Overcoming Common Problems

Coping with Type 2 Diabetes

Susan Elliot-Wright

sheldon PRESS

First published in Great Britain in 2005

Sheldon Press
36 Causton Street
London SW1P 4ST

Copyright © Susan Elliot-Wright 2005

The author and publisher have made every effort to ensure that the external
website and email addresses included in this book are correct and up to date
at the time of going to press. The author and publisher are not responsible
for the content, quality or continuing accessibility of the sites.

British Library Cataloguing-in-Publication Data
A catalogue record for this book is available from the British Library

ISBN-13: 978–0–85969–961–7
ISBN-10: 0–85969–961–7

1 3 5 7 9 10 8 6 4 2

Typeset by Deltatype Limited, Birkenhead, Merseyside
Printed in Great Britain by
Ashford Colour Press

Overcoming Common Problems Series

Overcoming Common Problems Series

Contents

Acknowledgements

I would like to thank all those who were kind enough to share with me their experiences of type 2 diabetes, and also those individuals and organizations who helped me to get my facts straight, in particular Diabetes UK who patiently answered my many, many questions.

Introduction

The full name for diabetes, diabetes mellitus, has Greek and Latin roots. 'Diabetes' comes from a Greek word meaning 'to siphon' or 'to flow through', and 'mellitus' comes from a Latin word meaning 'honey-sweet'. There are two different types of diabetes – type 1 and type 2. Although this book does look briefly at type 1, it is concerned primarily with type 2, which is the most common. As it is rather cumbersome to refer to 'type 2 diabetes' throughout the text, the term 'diabetes' is used often, and it may refer to both types or to type 2 only (but not to type 1 only).

You may be reading this book because you have type 2 diabetes yourself, or because someone close to you has been diagnosed with the disease. Alternatively, you may be in what is considered to be a high-risk group and want to know more about the prevention side of things. Whatever your reason for approaching the subject, this book should provide an insight into the condition and its causes, as well as plenty of advice on how to reduce your risk of developing diabetes and how to keep it under control if you do.

While Chapter 1 looks closely at what diabetes is, some readers may prefer to turn first to Chapter 2 which is about coping with diagnosis. This may be useful even if it is not you that has been diagnosed. It looks at how a diagnosis can affect people and the sort of stages they might go through after hearing they have the disease.

You'll probably want to dip in and out of the text according to the particular chapters or areas that interest you. But a word of caution: if you turn straight to the chapter on complications (Chapter 4), you're quite likely to scare yourself witless as you read the more alarming and gruesome bits about heart attacks, kidney failure, gangrene and amputation. So do please remember that it is perfectly possible to have type 2 diabetes and lead a normal, healthy and fulfilling life.

The prevalence of type 2 diabetes is increasing with alarming rapidity. Around 2 million people in the UK now have diabetes, compared with 1.4 million in 1996. In 90–95 per cent of cases, this will be type 2. Experts are talking about a diabetes 'epidemic', predicting a staggering three million cases by 2010, and the picture is similar in many countries across the world. So what has caused this global surge in the disease? It is no coincidence that the other condition reaching epidemic levels in developed countries is obesity. This is not to say that everyone who has type 2 diabetes is obese or even overweight, but it is one of the main contributory factors. We look at this and other possible causes in more detail in Chapter 3.

Although diabetes has been around for a very long time, the increased number of people with type 2 does seem to be a modern phenomenon, with our refined diets and more sedentary lifestyles contributing to the weight gain that is often associated with the disease. In order to develop diabetes, you need to have the 'diabetes gene', but some experts suggest that there's strong link between genetic and environmental factors. Our hunter-gatherer ancestors had a 'survival gene', which helped them to store surplus energy as abdominal fat during periods of starvation. When exposed to the sedentary lifestyle and the high-sugar and high-fat diets of the twenty-first century, these genes carry on storing energy as fat, only there are no longer any periods of starvation so the person is then predisposed to obesity, insulin resistance and type 2 diabetes. This is known as the 'thrifty-gene hypothesis' – described as '. . . a collision between thrifty genes and an affluent society'.

In many cases, type 2 diabetes can be controlled with diet and exercise alone, and you as the patient will play a major role in managing your treatment. Chapters 5 and 6 look in detail at how you can use diet and exercise to treat your condition or, if you're in a high-risk group, to prevent or delay its onset. Type 2 diabetes is one of the few diseases where the patient plays a major role it its treatment, so learning about the illness is vital. But be careful how you do your research. Not everything you read has been scrupu-lously researched, and some things are just plain inaccurate, leading many people to have rather strange ideas about the illness. Chapter 10 is an at-a-glance guide to some of the myths you may come across.

Although many people manage to control their diabetes with diet and exercise for a long period, they may need some form of medication eventually, and some will need to take insulin. Chapter 7 looks in detail at a range of diabetes drugs and at when and why they might be prescribed. We also look at insulin and how it's used.

There is no doubt that having type 2 diabetes will have a major effect on your life. Chapter 9 looks at some of the emotional and psychological difficulties you may have to face, such as depression and sexual difficulties. It also covers practical considerations, such as to cope with your illness while travelling abroad, how it may affect your job, your ability to drive and so on. Inevitably, there will be some negative effects of any illness, but hopefully learning more about your condition will help you to deal with and maybe even overcome these. There may also be positive things about having type 2 diabetes (although you'll probably find that hard to believe if you've just been diagnosed) and we look at these in Chapter 9 as well.

Having any incurable illness is frightening, but the more you understand about that illness and its treatment, the less scary it will seem. In the case of many conditions, you have to rely entirely on your doctors for your treatment and this makes you feel out of control. With type 2 diabetes, although you'll need advice and guidance at first, you'll probably be able to manage your illness yourself to a large extent, and this in itself is empowering, making the whole thing less terrifying. In reading this book, you're taking the first step towards educating yourself about your condition; and remember, knowledge is power!

1

What is type 2 diabetes?

Diabetes occurs as a result of a build up of glucose (sugar) in the blood. We need glucose to survive. It is an essential fuel, enabling the brain to function properly, the heart to pump blood around the body, and the muscles to move around and control breathing and so on. But it is important to keep the levels right: too much or too little and we become ill. None at all and we'd die.

When we eat something, the digestive system immediately sets about breaking it down into sugars and other components that can be effectively used by the body for fuel, growth and repair. The main sugar is glucose, which passes through the wall of the gut and into your bloodstream. After a meal, your blood glucose level begins to rise and your pancreas, a gland that sits just behind your stomach, secretes the hormone insulin. Insulin acts as a sort of facilitator for the body, taking glucose from the bloodstream and carrying it into the cells and tissues, which are able to use it as fuel.

Some of the glucose is converted into glycogen and stored by the body, mainly in the liver and muscles, for use when levels fall between meals. As glucose levels fall, so does the secretion of insulin. Some of the glycogen is then converted back into glucose and released into the bloodstream, triggering the production of more insulin, and so on.

When there is a shortage of insulin, the body cannot use the glucose properly and, as a result, the glucose builds up in the blood. The body then struggles to rid itself of the excess glucose, causing the kidneys to work overtime as they try to flush out the syrupy substance and consequently produce two of the most common symptoms of diabetes – the frequent need to pass urine and the thirst that results from the loss of fluid.

What's the difference between type 1 and type 2?

Type 1 diabetes is much less common than type 2 and is usually, though not always, associated with children and teenagers. In fact it used to be called juvenile diabetes or early-onset diabetes. Another term that is sometimes still used is insulin-dependent diabetes mellitus (IDDM). The main difference is that type 1 is an autoimmune disorder – where the body appears to turn against itself – whereas type 2 is mainly due to what is known as insulin resistance, of which more later.

In type 1 diabetes, the immune system attacks insulin-producing cells in the pancreas, called beta cells, having mistakenly recognized them as invading organisms. Consequently, the body produces less and less insulin until eventually, when most of the beta cells have been destroyed, the symptoms of diabetes become obvious and the person is given insulin treatment. Someone with type 1 will need insulin injections for the rest of his or her life, simply because the body is no longer able to make its own insulin. Type 1 diabetes is often diagnosed between the ages of 11 and 16 and rarely after age 30, although it can appear at any age.

In type 2, the pancreas still produces insulin, but for some reason it just doesn't work properly. This is known as insulin resistance. Imagine the insulin as a key, opening up the doors of the cells to allow the glucose in. If you are insulin resistant, it's as though the key is bent or broken and won't turn in the lock. The majority of people with type 2 diabetes produce a normal amount of insulin but have insulin resistance. A small number simply don't produce enough insulin to meet the body's requirements.

If you have insulin resistance, your body will usually realize this and start frantically producing more insulin to compensate. After a while, the insulin-producing cells in the pancreas become worn out and are unable to keep up effective production. This is known as beta-cell failure. As a result, your blood glucose level rises and this is when you're likely to be diagnosed with diabetes.

Type 2 diabetes is still sometimes known as non-insulin-dependent diabetes mellitus (NIDDM). It used to be called mature-onset diabetes or, less sensitively, old-age diabetes, and indeed it was usually associated with older people, but in the twenty-first century, more and more younger people are being diagnosed.

What are the symptoms?

One of the scary things about type 2 diabetes is that you can have it for months or even years before you know you have it – unlike type

1, which tends to come on quite suddenly as more and more insulin-producing cells are destroyed. The symptoms can be mild and cause so little trouble that you put it down to being 'under the weather'. But undiagnosed diabetes is extremely dangerous because the excess glucose can damage the nerves and cause all sorts of serious health complications including heart disease, stroke or even blindness. This is why it's so important to be aware of the disease and its symptoms, especially if you are in a high-risk group.

Often the first noticeable symptom is *an increased need to pass urine*. But this can be easily missed. If you're around middle age or older, you might put it down to age. If you're a woman you'll probably put it down to the fact that you've had kids. But finding that you need to go to the loo frequently, at night as well as during the day, could be a sign that your kidneys are working extra hard. Passing large amounts of urine leads to dehydration, which leads to thirst. You then need to replace all that fluid you're losing so you drink more – another common early symptom.

Other symptoms include:

- *Blurred vision* – this can be due to an excess of glucose in the tissues of the eye, in which case reducing blood glucose levels can improve vision. Or it may be due to retinopathy (see Chapter 4) a complication of diabetes in which high blood glucose has actually damaged the eye. If this is the case, the damage can be halted but not reversed.
- *Tiredness and fatigue* – this occurs because the body is unable to move glucose from the bloodstream into the cells so that it can be utilized as energy
- *Recurrent infections* – skin infections such as spots or boils, yeast infections such as thrush, and slow healing of cuts or grazes. Such recurrent infections are due to reduced immune function as a result of high glucose levels in the blood.
- *Itchy skin*, especially around the genitals.
- *Tingling or pins and needles in the hands or feet* – this can happen when the nerves have been irritated by the excess glucose.

How is type 2 diabetes diagnosed?

Some cases of diabetes are discovered after a routine test arouses the doctor's suspicions – high levels of glucose in your urine, for example, would lead your doctor to investigate further. Some people are advised to see their doctor by their optician after a routine eye check reveals changes in the blood vessels in the eye suggesting a possible complication of diabetes. But for most people, it is a combination of discovering they may be at risk (see Chapter 3) and noticing changes that could be symptoms of diabetes that sends them to the doctor in the first instance. If you suspect you may have diabetes, don't delay discussing this with your doctor. The sooner diabetes is diagnosed, the sooner treatment and control can begin, and the less likely it is that complications will arise or long-term damage will occur.

Linda, aged 49, noticed her eyesight deteriorating quite rapidly. She bought a pair of reading glasses and used a magnifying glass whenever she had to check a map or read the label on a can of beans. But her sight was getting progressively worse, so after a while she made an appointment to see her optician. She noticed the examination took longer than usual but was surprised when he suggested she see her doctor to be tested for diabetes. 'He'd noticed some changes in my eyes that he thought could indicate diabetes. The doctor then referred me to the hospital for blood tests and, sure enough, I was diagnosed with type 2 diabetes. I was totally shocked at first, but the more I think about it, the more I realize there had been other symptoms; I just hadn't taken much notice. I'd been getting up to go to the toilet three or four times a night but like the eyesight thing, I just put it down to age. It was a terrible shock to be told I had type 2 diabetes, but at least now I know, so I'm doing all I can to get it under control.'

What type of testing is available?

Your doctor will make a diagnosis after looking at your symptoms and carrying out tests to measure your blood glucose levels. Many doctors have blood glucose meters in their surgeries and can carry out an on the spot test by taking a tiny drop of blood from a finger prick. However, these meters are not as accurate as laboratory tests so your doctor will probably recommend further testing to confirm the diagnosis.

The level of glucose in your blood varies throughout the day. A blood sample taken first thing in the morning before breakfast would give what is called your 'fasting glucose'. You will be asked to fast overnight or for at least eight hours, possibly longer, before the test. You can also be tested when you haven't been fasting, and the result is known as your 'random glucose'. This test can be taken at any time but, although it takes into account that you will probably have eaten recently, it is not as reliable as the fasting blood glucose test. Both these tests may be carried out on two different days just to confirm the findings. A fasting glucose concentration of more than 7 millimoles per litre (mmol/l) or a random glucose of more than 11.1 mmol/l would indicate that you have diabetes.

Sometimes, even these tests are not clear and a further test is needed. The most accurate type of testing is the oral glucose tolerance test (OGTT), which measures how good your body is at dealing with glucose. It may be recommended if your fasting blood glucose results are borderline – higher than normal but not high enough for a diagnosis of diabetes. Your glucose levels will be measured when you arrive for the test after fasting, you'll be given a drink containing around 75 grams of glucose. Your blood glucose levels will be measured again two hours later. As with the random blood glucose test, a level of 11.0 mmol/l or higher will confirm diabetes. A level of more than 7.8 mmol/l but less than 11.0 mmol/l indicates impaired glucose tolerance (IGT). A level of less than 7.8 mmol/l but more than 6.0 mmol/l indicates impaired fasting glycaemia (IFG). Both IGT and IFG are often referred to as 'pre-diabetes', although this does not necessarily mean you will go on to develop diabetes.

What if I have pre-diabetes?

Pre-diabetes does not mean you have diabetes or 'borderline diabetes' – experts say there is no such thing – and therefore you are not currently at risk of the complications of diabetes. However, if you have IGT, you may be more at risk of heart disease, and an increased risk of developing type 2 diabetes is associated with both IGT and IFG. If your tests show that you have IGT or IFG, try to see it as an early warning system – your body is telling you that it is having difficulty processing glucose. It's often the case that those with IGT or IFG have a sedentary lifestyle, eat a diet that's not very healthy and are a little (or a lot) overweight. Now is the time to be honest with yourself. Could you be overweight? Do you take enough exercise? Maybe your diet could be improved. Making a few slight changes (see Chapter 5) could significantly reduce your risk of developing type 2 diabetes. It will also help to reduce your risk of heart disease and, what's more, you'll feel happier and healthier in general. Even if you make these changes, of course, you can't completely eradicate the risk so you should ask your doctor to test your blood glucose every few years.

2

Coping with diagnosis

Most people find their diagnosis comes as a shock, especially as it often comes to light by accident, either as the result of a routine test or while another health problem is being investigated. It can be difficult to come to terms with the fact that you have, or that someone close to you has, a serious, incurable disease, but incurable doesn't mean terminal, nor does it mean uncontrollable. As you will see from the rest of the book, with the right information and support, many people with type 2 diabetes are able to control their condition and stay fit, healthy and active for a great many years. For some people, diabetes management may be more difficult, owing to factors beyond their control. Others already have serious health problems as a result of their diabetes by the time they are diagnosed. But whatever your own situation, bear in mind that two positive things have already happened:

- The diagnosis has been made. This means that you and your health-care team can start taking action immediately to get your blood glucose levels under control and reduce the risks to your health.
- You are reading this book, which means you're already taking steps to gather information about the condition so that you can manage it in the best way possible.

Reaction and acceptance

You may experience a series of very strong emotions when you're first diagnosed. It's not uncommon to feel anger, guilt, grief and even fear, and your mind will be buzzing with questions, the first of which will probably be, 'why me?' It may or may not be possible to answer that question. It may be that you have several of the risk factors mentioned in Chapter 3. For example, if you have a parent, an uncle and two siblings with the disease, you're over 50 and you're carrying more than a few spare pounds, you may have already considered the possibility of developing the disease. But you may have none of the obvious risk factors and still be diagnosed, in which case it's slightly more difficult to explain. One thing to bear in mind is: it's not your fault. If it's anyone's fault, it's that of your ancestors, because in order to develop diabetes, you must have diabetic genes. If you don't have the genes, you could eat chocolate and candy floss all day, scoff burgers and chips on a regular basis, do no exercise and still not get diabetes. However, you can also have the genes and not develop the illness. For example, if you lived in a country where food was scarce and you ate a frugal, unrefined diet to sustain your long days of physical labour, chances are you wouldn't get diabetes.

Whether you can trace your diabetes to known risk factors or whether it appears to have come out of the blue, you are bound to feel angry that you have developed the illness. Allow yourself to feel angry – you have a right to be seriously annoyed! But try not to let your anger take over and, more importantly, don't let it get in the way of the action you can take to improve your health.

When you've just been diagnosed, it's easy to blame yourself. You'll probably think, if only I hadn't eaten so much red meat, drunk so much beer, smoked so many cigarettes! Or, if only I'd gone to the gym or eaten more fruit or walked to the office! And so on and so forth. Everyone who is diagnosed with any serious illness wonders whether they could have done something to prevent it, and the answer is: possibly, but probably not. And if you hadn't done whatever you think may have led to your diabetes, what about all the other less-than-perfectly-healthy things that most of us do, most of the time? Even if you had lived an active life of dietary perfection, you may still have got diabetes. The important thing is that you now know, and you can start to fight it. Diabetes is one of the few serious conditions that you really can help to control yourself, preferably with plenty of support from your diabetes healthcare team.

After 'why me?', you'll probably think, 'Perhaps they made a mistake'. Well, perhaps they did, but it's unlikely. Hoping the diagnosis is wrong is a common reaction, and it's easier than accepting the truth. After all, you're being asked to acknowledge that you have an incurable disease and that the pattern of your life is going to change from now on. Will you still be able to enjoy your favourite foods? Will you have to go back and forth to the doctor or hospital every five minutes? Are you going to end up sticking needles in yourself? How will your family and friends react when you tell them that you're 'a diabetic'? A day, an hour, even a minute before your diagnosis, these were things you didn't have to think about, so naturally it's tempting to want to deny what you've been told, to refuse to accept it. But accept it you must. Don't waste time and energy blaming yourself or fantasizing that they got your blood sample mixed up with someone else's. You've got diabetes and it's bad luck, but the sooner you are able to accept your diagnosis, the quicker you can start learning about the condition, taking control and managing the situation.

It's common to feel a sense of grief after you've been diagnosed. This is also perfectly normal. You have, in a sense, suffered a loss. You're grieving the life that you would – or might – have had if you hadn't got diabetes, the person you may have been had you not got an illness that is clearly going to demand a lot of your time and attention. You may also feel afraid, nervous and anxious about your illness. This is perfectly normal. You may know very little, if anything, about diabetes when you're first diagnosed, and the unknown is always more frightening than the familiar. Some doctors can be less than tactful in breaking the news and that certainly doesn't help you towards calm acceptance. But by arming yourself with as much knowledge and information as possible, you are not only taking the first steps to managing your illness, you will also feel considerably more in control and this will help you feel less afraid.

Thinking about the future

There's no denying that controlling diabetes will take a fair bit of time and effort on your part and on that of those close to you, especially while you're still learning about the disease. But as you and your loved ones become more knowledgeable, you'll find you're having to spend less time thinking about your illness and more time simply living your life. Managing type 2 diabetes is time-intensive, and it can be tempting to think, 'Well, I've got it anyway, so why waste time reading about diets and testing and levels and so on?' What you need to bear in mind is that, even if you feel reasonably OK at the moment, type 2 diabetes is a progressive illness. The progression is slow, it's true – and that means you have time to act – but it will not get better on its own. Untreated, it will get worse, increasing your risk of serious, even life-threatening consequences. It is now widely acknowledged that good diabetes care depends largely on patient knowledge and understanding – in other words, this is one disease you can't leave to the doctors! Every time you find yourself thinking it's too much effort, remember that the benefits of taking control are immediate and long-lasting. Even if you were not aware of any obvious symptoms, you'll find that the tiniest of adjustments to your diet and lifestyle will give you more energy and make you feel fitter in general. And if you have been suffering some of the unpleasant symptoms we looked at in Chapter 1, bringing your blood glucose levels under control will quickly improve your condition, and those symptoms will start to improve.

3

What causes type 2 diabetes?

Around five per cent of the world's population has diabetes. There are around two million people with diabetes in the UK and over 18 million in the USA, the vast majority – around 90 per cent – have type 2 diabetes. The figures are rising year upon year. It is thought that by 2010 the UK figure will have risen to three million, while a study published in the *Journal of the American Medical Association* in 2003 predicted that, if the rate of diabetes continues to increase, one in three Americans born in 2000 will be diagnosed with diabetes by the year 2050.

Worryingly, experts believe that for every person who has been diagnosed with type 2 diabetes, there is another as yet unaware that he or she has the condition. According to Diabetes UK, a staggering half of all those with type 2 diabetes already have some complications of the disease by the time they are diagnosed.

Why is it on the increase?

A combination of reasons is thought to be responsible for the increase in type 2 diabetes, including lack of exercise, increasing reliance on convenience or take-away meals and poor diet in general. The risk of developing type 2 diabetes increases for those who are overweight or have sedentary lifestyles, and it is 10 times greater for those who are clinically obese. Like type 2 diabetes, obesity is also increasing, especially in the UK, which, with 22 per cent of adults now classified as obese compared with 14 per cent 10 years ago, has the fastest growing rate of obesity in the developed world. In the USA, a third of adults are overweight or obese. It is also true that modern-day living increases stress and leaves us with little time to attend to our health. It may be that as a consequence of this, warning signs are being ignored whereas, if they'd been picked up, a change in diet and lifestyle might have been enough to prevent diabetes from developing.

Who is at risk?

There are a number of risk factors involved in type 2 diabetes, so let's look at them separately.

Overweight and obesity

Excess body weight is a major risk factor in type 2 diabetes, with around 80 per cent of people with diabetes being overweight at diagnosis. According to the World Health Organization, a healthy body mass index (BMI) range is from 18 to 25. You are said to be obese if your BMI is greater than 30. The BMI is simply a way of working out whether you are the right weight for your height. To work out your BMI, measure your height in metres and multiply the figure by itself, then weigh yourself in kilograms and divide the weight by the height squared (your height multiplied by itself). So for example, if you're 1.7 metres tall and weigh 68 kilograms, the calculation would be: $1.7 \times 1.7 = 2.89$, then $68 \div 2.89 = 23.52$. So your BMI would be 23.52

Another way of doing this is to weigh yourself in pounds, multiply the figure by 703, divide it by your height in inches and then divide it by your height in inches a second time. Therefore, if you're 5 feet 6 inches (i.e. 66 inches) and weigh 150 pounds, the calculation would be:

$150 \times 703 = 105,450 \div 66 \div 66 = 24.20$. So your BMI would be 24.20.

It is thought that over-eating puts extra stress on the insides of individual cells in the body. When the membrane inside the cell has more nutrients to process than it can deal with, it sends out an 'alarm' signal, which tells the insulin receptors on the cell surface to dampen down their action. This results in insulin resistance, which leads to high concentrations of the sugar glucose in the blood.

Abdominal obesity

Your shape also has a bearing on your risk of developing diabetes. Central body fat – being overweight and 'apple shaped', that is, where the extra weight is stored around the middle rather than evenly distributed or stored around the hips and thighs – is strongly associated with insulin resistance and increased risk of diabetes and cardiovascular disease. If you are a man and your waist measures more than 40 inches (102 centimetres) or if you are a woman and your waist measures more than 35 inches (88 centimetres), your risk of developing these conditions could be significantly increased.

Gestational diabetes/large baby

If you give birth to a baby weighing 9 pounds or more at birth, or if you have gestational diabetes during your pregnancy, you are more likely to develop type 2 diabetes later, even though gestational diabetes usually disappears after the baby is born. You will also be more at risk if your mother had gestational diabetes while she was expecting you.

Family history

Your genetic make up has a strong bearing on whether or not you are likely to develop type 2 diabetes, although even if you have the genes, there also needs to be some environmental trigger, such as lack of exercise or poor diet, to kick start the action of the genes. In general, if a family member has either type 1 or type 2, you are at increased risk, with the risk being greater the closer the relative. It is also possible to have diabetes even if you have no family history.

As a rough guide:

- If both your parents have the condition, your risk of developing it is around 75 per cent
- If one parent or a sibling has it, your risk is 15 per cent
- For non-identical twins, your risk is 10 per cent
- And if your identical twin has it, your risk is 90 per cent

Ethnicity

For some reason, your risk of developing type 2 diabetes is significantly higher than that of the general population (between 3 and 5 per cent) if you are from a South Asian, black Caribbean or black African background. You are also more likely to diagnosed with the condition at a younger age.

The highest levels of diabetes are found in the Pima Indians of Arizona, where half of the adult population who live on US reservations has it. Around 70 per cent of children born to Pima mothers who had diabetes while they were pregnant go on to develop it themselves by the age of 25–34 years. While there certainly appears to be a genetic predisposition to type 2 diabetes among Pimas, environmental factors must also be taken into consideration. Even though they have the same genes as those living on the reservations, Pima Indians who choose to stay in the mountains of Mexico where they tend to have a more physically demanding lifestyle, have a much lower rate of diabetes, with only one in 15 developing it.

Age

In general, you are more at risk of type 2 diabetes if you are over 40 and that risk increases further as you get older. However, while it used to be relatively uncommon to see type 2 in those under 40, it is now becoming more prevalent. In the UK, almost 100,000 people aged 15–44 have type 2 diabetes, and while the number of children under 14 with the disease is still fairly low, this too is on the increase, especially in the UK and USA, where obesity levels are rising quite dramatically. In the early 1990s the average age of diagnosis was 52. A recent US study suggests it is now 46.

Children with type 2 diabetes

Doctors are seeing more and more adolescents with type 2 diabetes. There are currently no accurate figures in the UK but there are thought to be at least 100 and possibly up to 1,500 children with the disease. The increase in the US is being described as an 'epidemic', with roughly four times as many children being diagnosed in 2002–2003 as in the early 1990s, which was when doctors first began to see cases of type 2 in children – usually overweight children with overweight parents.

Although there have been cases as young as six, children who develop type 2 diabetes often do so around puberty. Changes in hormone levels during this period can affect the action of insulin and can cause insulin resistance. In children this is often indicated by a skin condition called acanthosis nigricans, which results in velvety, dirty-looking dark patches around the neck and other skin folds. Other symptoms in children are similar to those in adults – frequent urination and thirst (although this may not be as severe as in adults), blurred vision, tiredness and slow healing of cuts and grazes. Obesity is a significant factor in children and teenagers with type 2 diabetes, and as children become increasingly inactive and eat more sugary or

17

high-fat snacks and processed foods, the problem of obesity also increases.

There is some disagreement as to the definition of obesity in children, and calculating a child's BMI is much more complex than in adults because their BMI changes with age and there are differences between boys and girls. Your health visitor, doctor or paediatrician will have been keeping a record of your child's growth, including weight and height, since birth. The measurements are plotted on a percentile chart which gives an indication of how your child's weight and height compares with his or her peers. The 50th percentile is the median line, so if your child's BMI fell exactly on that line, it would mean that half of the other boys or girls of the same age in the country are lighter, and half are heavier. If it fell on the 70th percentile, it means 30 per cent of his or her peers are heavier, and 70 per cent do not weigh as much. As a very rough guide, a BMI on the 85th percentile would indicate some concern and risk of overweight. A BMI on the 90th percentile is considered overweight and above the 98th percentile would be considered obese. It must be stressed that this is a rough guide – your child's BMI should be calculated and interpreted by a medical practitioner.

Pre-diabetes

If you have impaired glucose tolerance (IGT) or impaired fasting glycaemia (IFG), both of which may also be known as pre-diabetes, it doesn't mean that you'll definitely develop the disease, but it does mean that your blood glucose levels are higher than they should be. This means you're at increased risk, both of developing diabetes and of developing cardiovascular disease.

Syndrome X

Syndrome X is a relatively new term, coined by an endocrinologist (someone who specializes in problems with endocrine glands such as the pancreas) in the late 1980s, for a collection of symptoms that would suggest someone is at fairly high risk of developing diabetes. This group of symptoms is also known as metabolic syndrome. Originally, a diagnosis of syndrome X would depend on four main symptoms:

- Insulin resistance
- Abdominal obesity – being disproportionately fat around the middle
- High levels of triglycerides (the chemical form of some fats) and low levels of high-density lipoproteins (HDL) – 'good' cholesterol)
- High blood pressure

These days, doctors are more inclined to take into account other symptoms, and may look at your family history and your diet and lifestyle as well as carrying out blood tests to check such things as your levels of blood glucose, triglycerides and cholesterol. You can get a rough idea of how likely you are to have syndrome X by looking at the following questions:

- Do you find it impossible to lose weight?
- Are you 'apple shaped' (i.e. do you tend to put on weight around the middle)?
- Are you constantly hungry, even soon after eating?
- Do you crave or eat a lot of carbohydrates, such as bread, pasta, pizzas, cereal and cakes?
- Do you have high blood pressure?
- Do you have problems with cholesterol?
- Do you have blood glucose problems?
- Does any close member of your family have diabetes?

If you answer yes to three or more of these questions, you may well be diagnosed with syndrome X. The main cause of syndrome X is raised insulin levels due to insulin resistance, which is thought to be influenced largely by diet. For example, it has been noted that some ethnic groups, such as Native Americans and Hawaiians, who are at relatively high risk of developing insulin resistance and diabetes, only became so when they started eating a diet rich in refined sugars and carbohydrates.

Humans were originally designed to live off high quantities of plant foods and small amounts of meat. Our 'hunter-gatherer' ancestors lived on vegetation and fairly low-fat meat – game meat is lean and lower in saturated fat. Then we began developing agriculture and, in particular, cultivating grains. But we're not designed to chew grains properly, so they have to be crushed, a process that immediately refines them and makes large amounts of carbohydrates available for digestion. We have continued to change our diets, refining and processing even more and moving even further away from our evolutionary baseline diet. We now consume vast amounts of refined carbohydrates in such foods as pasta, breads, cereals and breakfast bars. Many foods are now fried in refined oils or contain partially hydrogenated oils (vegetable oils processed so that they have some characteristics of saturated fats). Many foods also contain large amounts of sugar, and often, very few nutrients.

This sort of diet causes huge problems with glucose and insulin levels. Refined sugars and carbohydrates rapidly boost glucose levels. In order to reduce theses levels, the pancreas secretes large amounts of insulin to help transport glucose into the muscles or liver. Over time, these raised levels of insulin overwhelm the insulin receptors on the cells. Eventually, these cells become resistant or insensitive to insulin, and blood levels of glucose and insulin rise, increasing the risk of syndrome X, type 2 diabetes and other conditions such as heart disease.

Can type 2 diabetes be prevented?

A number of studies have looked into whether people who are at risk of type 2 diabetes can actually be helped to prevent it from developing, and there is significant evidence to suggest that this is possible. Experts agree that lifestyle changes can, at the very least, delay the onset of the disease, if not prevent it altogether.

In 2001, a major clinical trial that supports this was completed in the USA. The Diabetes Prevention Program (DPP) was designed to find the most effective ways of preventing type 2 diabetes in overweight people with pre-diabetes. The study, which involved 3,234 people with IGT, all of whom had a BMI of 25 or more, divided volunteers into three groups:

- The first group took up moderate exercise – typically 30 minutes' walking, five days a week – and reduced their intake of calories of fat.
- Volunteers in the second group were treated with metformin, an

oral diabetes drug that lowers blood glucose levels by reducing the over-production of glucose in the liver.
- Those in the control group were given placebo pills in place of metformin, and, like the second group, were also given standard medical information and advice on diet and exercise.

Researchers found that the first group, who lost around 5 to 7 per cent of their body weight through diet and exercise, reduced their risk of diabetes by 58 per cent. This lifestyle intervention worked equally well in men and women and in all ethnic groups; however, it was particularly effective in people over 60, who reduced their risk by an impressive 71 per cent. Also, many of the volunteers in this group found that their blood glucose levels returned to normal.

There was some lowering of risk in the metformin group, whose members had a 38 per cent lower incidence of type 2 diabetes. However, although metformin was effective in all the ethnic groups and in both men and women, it was less effective in older volunteers and in those who were less overweight.

As a result of the DPP, America launched 'Small steps, big rewards', a national diabetes prevention campaign aimed at raising awareness of just how effective even moderate changes to diet and lifestyle can be in preventing or delaying the onset of type 2 diabetes.

We'll go into much more detail about how diabetes can be prevented in Chapter 5, but, in general, eating a healthy diet, not allowing your body mass index to rise above 25, and getting regular exercise will help. If you are already overweight or have high blood glucose levels, now is the time to take action. Losing weight, getting your blood pressure down and lowering your cholesterol levels will all help lower the risk of complications from high blood glucose levels.

Can certain illnesses or medicines increase risk?

Women who have polycystic ovary syndrome are at increased risk if they are overweight. Some drugs, such as steroids, can raise blood glucose, and diabetes may be diagnosed. However, it is not certain that steroids actually cause the diabetes, or whether their effect simply unmasks the disease in someone who is already susceptible. Very occasionally, diabetes develops as a result of damage to the pancreas by high doses of steroid-based anti-rejection drugs given to organ transplant patients. Some protease inhibitors (used in the treatment of HIV) and some anti-psychotics are also thought to cause diabetes, although again this is not entirely certain. There are also a number of drugs that raise blood glucose levels, even in people without diabetes, but this usually resolves once the drug is discontinued.

4

Long-term complications and foot problems

Diabetes is often thought of as a fairly minor illness. After all, millions of people have is and seem to survive, right? Well, it's certainly true that diabetes can be controlled and that someone can have the disease and lead a relatively normal life. However, undiagnosed or uncontrolled diabetes can lead to a number of serious, even life-threatening complications.

Cardiovascular disease

Cardiovascular disease, which includes both stroke and coronary heart disease, is one of the commonest long-term complications of diabetes. If you have diabetes, you're five times more likely to develop cardiovascular disease than the general population. It's the biggest cause of premature death in people with diabetes, accounting for around 80 per cent of deaths, and what's really worrying is that more than half of those with type 2 diabetes have some evidence of CVD by the time they are diagnosed.

Cardovascular disease occurs as a result of a blockage in the arteries, caused by a process known as atherosclerosis, which can be accelerated by diabetes. This can cause stroke when the blood vessels serving the brain are affected, and coronary heart disease when the coronary (heart) arteries are affected. Arteriosclerosis is the term given to the thickening and hardening of the arteries, which can occur for a number of reasons including ageing, high blood pressure and diabetes. Atherosclerosis is a type of arteriosclerosis, and is characterized by the build up of plaque – a combination of cholesterol and other fatty matter, calcium and various other blood components – on the inner arterial walls. A hard shell or scar covers the plaque and the artery wall thus thickens, loses its elasticity, and becomes jagged with plaque instead of smooth.

The thickened arterial wall means that blood flow is decreased because there is a much narrower space for the blood to move through. This poor circulation can cause some of the other complications addressed in this chapter. Narrowed arteries also make blockage more likely, and if the plaques rupture, causing the sudden formation of blood clots, there is a danger that they will block the artery completely, causing heart attack or stroke.

You can help prevent cardiovascular problems by keeping an eye on your blood pressure, reducing the saturated fat, salt and cholesterol in your diet, losing weight and taking more exercise – more on this in Chapter 6. Above all, give up smoking! Stopping smoking needn't be agony, and you'll feel so much better so quickly, you'll wonder why you didn't do it years ago! There are a number of ways to give up smoking, and there are various products and services available, all claiming various success rates. Some of these can certainly help you to stop, but they can't do it for you, so you need to make a mental commitment to giving up. Prescription anti-smoking medicines are not suitable for everyone, but it may be worth asking your doctor about these. Or you may want to try nicotine replacement therapy (such as nicotine patches, nicotine chewing gum, inhalers). Some people respond well to anti-smoking clinics, self-help groups and support lines – studies show that quitters who have support are more successful. Or, if you prefer a do-it-yourself approach, there are a number of self-help books available (see Further reading, page 113).

Diabetic nephropathy (diabetic kidney disease)

Kidney disease occurs as a result of damage, often over many years, to blood vessels in the glomeruli (the filtering unit of the kidney). It can lead to kidney failure and even death. Around a third of all those with diabetes will develop kidney disease, with the risk increasing with the duration of the diabetes – 25 years after being diagnosed with type 1 or type 2, the risk of developing kidney disease is 40–50 per cent.

After we've digested a meal, the various substances pass into the blood and are transported in the bloodstream for the body to use or to discard as waste. The kidneys contain millions of capillaries (small blood vessels), each full of tiny holes that act as filters. As blood flows through the capillaries, the waste products, which have been broken down into small molecules, pass through the holes to be expelled as urine while the more useful substances, such as protein, stay in the blood. When blood glucose levels are too high, the kidneys have to work extra hard to cope, and over the years the blood vessels become damaged. The result of this is that the filtering system becomes less efficient at removing waste and excess water from the body. Useful products such as protein begin to leak through into the urine and waste products start to build up in the blood. Having small amounts of protein in the urine is called microalbuminuria, while the presence of larger amounts is called macroalbuminuria. If nothing is done to halt the process, the kidneys will eventually fail altogether. This failure is known as end-stage renal disease (ESRD) and is very serious, causing the person to need to have their blood filtered artificially by machine – kidney dialysis – or to have a kidney transplant.

Unfortunately, symptoms of diabetic kidney disease may not be apparent until severe damage has occurred and kidney function is minimal or ceases completely. One of the first indications that the kidneys are failing tends to be a build up of fluid causing swelling of the body tissue (oedema). Other symptoms include nausea and vomiting, fatigue and poor appetite.

The best way to prevent diabetic kidney disease is to keep your blood glucose levels within the target range, as suggested by your diabetes care team. An ideal range is usually 4–7 mmol/l but in some cases – in older, frail people, for example – a higher upper limit of maybe 11 or 12 mmol/l may be appropriate. Research has shown that keeping blood glucose under control reduces the risk of microalbuminuria by a third, and in those who already have microalbuminuria, the risk of it progressing to macroalbuminuria is lowered by half.

Control of blood glucose is also a vital part of treatment, as is control of blood pressure – even a slight rise in blood pressure can hasten the progress of kidney disease, causing it to worsen quite quickly. There are certain drugs that can lower blood pressure, and your doctor may recommend these drugs, but there are important steps you can take immediately to help lower your blood pressure: give up smoking, avoid alcohol or use it very sparingly, lower your salt intake and control your weight with diet and exercise. See Chapters 5 and 6 for more on diet and exercise.

Eye problems

When blood glucose levels have been abnormally high for 10 years or more, most people begin to show signs of retinopathy, and around 20 per cent of people with type 2 diabetes already have some signs by the time they are diagnosed. For some reason, high levels of glucose in the blood cause capillaries to become fragile and leaky, and there may be slight damage quite early on which can be seen by an ophthalmologist. The retina is the part of the eye which records images and flashes them to the brain via the optic nerve. The first sign of retinopathy is often fatty deposits; another common first sign is tiny swellings in the capillaries called aneurysms, which can be seen on the retina at the back of the eye.

At this early stage, known as non-proliferative retinopathy, vision may still be perfectly normal and need no treatment, although it's important to keep blood glucose levels down and to have regular eye checks to make sure the disease isn't progressing. However, if fluid leaks into the macular area of the retina, it could cause the retina to become swollen. This swelling is known as macular oedema and the distortion of the retina may result in some loss of vision.

If blood glucose remains high over a number of years, the disease may progress to proliferative retinopathy, a much more serious form that can cause loss of vision. In proliferative retinopathy, the capillaries are so badly damaged that they can no longer move blood around efficiently and so they shut down. When the body, clever machine that it is, realizes that these blood vessels have stopped working, it starts trying to fix the problem by frantically making new ones. In some parts of the body this is a good thing, but in the eye, these new capillaries can themselves obstruct vision or, because they tend to be inferior and are extra-fragile, they can leak blood into the clear fluid (the vitreous humour) of the eye. This is called vitreous haemorrhage. If blood clots and scar tissue begins to form, this can pull the retina away from its attachments. This is called retinal detachment, a serious condition that can lead to blindness.

Fortunately, laser surgery can now be used to seal leaky capillaries to prevent them from growing and leaking, in a procedure called photocoagulation, which is uncomfortable but fairly quick and straightforward.

Glaucoma

Although anyone can get glaucoma, you're 40 per cent more likely to develop it if you have diabetes. Glaucoma is where the air pressure inside your eye is higher than it should be. This increased pressure can damage the blood vessels that supply the retina and the optic nerve – the nerve that tells the brain what the eye is seeing – causing loss of vision, often starting with decreased peripheral vision. If caught early enough, glaucoma can be controlled effectively with eye drops or other medication. Each time you have your eyes tested, remind your ophthalmologist or optician that you have diabetes and ask to have your intraocular pressures measured.

Acute glaucoma, caused by a sudden increase in pressure and a complete blocking of fluid draining from the eye, is a medical emergency and should be treated without delay. Symptoms include sudden, severe pain, decreased vision, seeing halos around lights, and nausea and vomiting.

Cataracts

Cataracts are when the lens of the eye becomes cloudy. In people with diabetes, this is likely to be due to changes in the proteins in the eye as a result of raised blood glucose levels. Vision becomes blurred and deteriorates as the cloudiness progresses. The other main symptom is sensitivity to glare. Anyone can get cataracts, although they most commonly occur in people aged 60 or over. In younger people, they are more common in those with diabetes, in whom they are likely to develop earlier and more quickly. Again, keeping control of blood glucose will help to prevent cataracts from forming and progressing, as will giving up smoking, taking an antioxidant supplement and protecting your eyes from bright sunlight. If loss of vision is great enough to affect your daily life, surgical cataract removal is relatively simple and takes about 20 minutes under local anaesthetic. Ultrasound is used to liquefy the lens, which is then drawn out through a tiny incision and replaced with a synthetic lens. The procedure is generally very successful and recovery is fast.

Neuropathy and nerve damage

Neuropathy is the overall term used to describe nerve damage, although different doctors classify neuropathies differently, which can be confusing. There are a number of causes of nerve damage, including nutritional deficiency and some immune disorders, but diabetes is the most common. Indeed, one of the commonest complications of diabetes is diabetic neuropathy, which occurs when persistent high blood glucose levels causes damage to the peripheral nerves (the nerves that go from the brain and spinal cord to the rest of the body) or to the blood vessels that supply them. There are three different types of peripheral nerves:

- Motor nerves – these nerves carry signals to the muscles that control movement, enabling us to walk, dance or unscrew the lid of the coffee jar.
- Sensory nerves – these nerves take messages to the brain about movement, shape, texture, temperature and also about pain, whether from sensors on the skin or from deeper in the body.
- Autonomic nerves – these nerves control unconscious functions such as breathing, heart rate, body temperature, blood pressure and digestive processes.

Sometimes only one nerve is affected, and this is called mononeuropathy. Where the damage affects several nerves, the condition is called polyneuropathy. A common type of neuropathy is compression mononeuropathy, where a single nerve is damaged either by restricted blood flow to the nerve as a direct result of diabetes or by being squashed where they pass through a tight tunnel or over a lump of bone. Although people without diabetes can suffer compression mononeuropathy, the nerves of people with diabetes are more prone to compression injury. Carpal tunnel syndrome, where the median nerve becomes compressed as it passes through a tunnel of bone in the wrist, is probably the most common type of compression mononeuropathy. It is often seen in people whose work or lifestyle means they make repeated hand movements, such as typing or knitting. It can cause numbness, tingling and pain in the hand, especially the thumb and middle fingers.

Michelle was only just coming to terms with her diagnosis of type 2 diabetes when she started to have problems with her hand and wrist. 'I work as a cook in a nursery school catering for 100 children every day. I've always loved cooking and I really enjoy coming up with new recipes for the kids. But a few weeks after I was diagnosed with diabetes, I started to get pins and needles in my hand. Then I found I was having problems at work. I'd be chopping an onion and I'd suddenly lose my grip on the knife, or I'd be whisking custard or something and then find I couldn't feel my hand properly. Sometimes it would just feel numb, sometimes there would be a tingling sensation and other times I'd get a pain in my wrist. I put up with it for a while, but then the pain got quite bad, especially at night. I'd have to get out of bed and walk around until it went off before I could get back to sleep. Also, I'd started dropping things at work, and you can't be dropping great saucepans full of hot food in a busy kitchen, so I went to my doctor. She said it was carpal tunnel syndrome and that, while it was possibly caused by my job – I use my hands all the time, chopping and peeling and so on – the fact that I had diabetes meant I was more likely to get it than someone doing the same job who doesn't have diabetes. She asked me how I was coping with keeping my blood glucose levels under control and said I've got to be really careful to keep an eye on them because, apparently, I'm particularly vulnerable to nerve damage now, and at least I could prevent things from getting worse. I promised I'd keep a better watch on things. She gave me a support splint for my wrist and said I need to rest it for a while. If that doesn't work, they can do an operation to release the nerves. In the meantime, I'm going to make a real effort to keep my blood glucose down. I know I need to be careful, and I need to lose some weight, but to be honest, working with food all day makes it very difficult. Getting this carpal tunnel syndrome has scared me a bit because it's shown me that high blood glucose can actually do real damage to the body. I know it sounds stupid, but I didn't really take it in before.'

Motor nerve neuropathy

Damage to the motor nerves causes weakening and, eventually, wasting of the muscles, although this type of neuropathy is fairly rare in diabetes.

Distal symmetric neuropathy

This is the most common form of neuropathy. It tends to strike both sides of the body, affecting most commonly the feet and legs and sometimes the hands. Symptoms include tingling, burning, numbness, pain and loss of sensation, including the inability to feel vibration – in diagnosing this type of neuropathy, your doctor may hold a tuning fork against part of your foot to see whether you are able to feel the vibration.

Autonomic neuropathy

Depending on which nerves are affected, autonomic neuropathy can interfere with a number of different functions. It can play havoc with your digestive system, causing constipation, diarrhoea, nausea and vomiting, or it can affect the nerves of the stomach, causing a feeling of excessive fullness after even small meals. It can prevent the bladder from functioning properly. Paralysis of the bladder is common in this type of neuropathy – the bladder fails to respond to pressure as it fills with urine, leading to inefficient or infrequent emptying. As a result, urine tends to stay in the bladder for too long, which can lead to urinary tract infections. Damage to the nerves supplying the blood vessels can affect blood pressure, causing you to feel dizzy when you stand up too quickly. This is because your blood pressure control system is less efficient and can't react to the body's change of position quickly enough. Damage to these nerves may also affect temperature regulation, because it is dilation of the small blood vessels (capillaries) that helps to cool the body. The result is that you may sweat more than usual, especially at night or while eating (known as 'gustatory sweating').

Men with diabetes are more likely to develop erectile dysfunction because of blood vessel and nerve damage caused from high blood glucose levels. You may be unable to achieve an erection at all, your erection may not be strong enough to allow intercourse or it may be that you're unable to maintain your erection. Stopping smoking, which constricts blood vessels, and keeping blood glucose under control are some of the ways to reduce risks of erectile problems, but if you do experience difficulties, do discuss this with your doctor because there are a number of possible treatments available. It is also very important to discuss this with your partner, because sexual difficulty is a problem for the couple, not just for the person experiencing the physical cause. Very often, sexual difficulties become a vicious circle: you're unable to get an erection (for whatever reason), therefore you feel embarrassed and inadequate, therefore you can't get an erection. It can be deeply frustrating when your body won't do what your brain is telling it to, and we'll look more closely at sexual problems and the psychological effects of diabetes in Chapter 9.

Foot problems

Foot problems in people with diabetes can occur either as a result of impaired blood flow to the feet caused by damaged blood vessels, or as a result of nerve damage resulting in loss of sensation, which can in turn cause minor injuries to go unnoticed until infection develops.

Foot ulcers

According to Diabetes UK, around one in 10 people with diabetes will develop a foot ulcer at some stage. An ulcer is an open sore where the skin tissue has broken down so badly that you can see the underlying tissue. Ulcers need to be treated immediately to prevent them from leading to gangrene, a very serious condition that can result in amputation or even death. Around 15 per cent of foot ulcers will result in amputation.

You are more prone to foot ulcers if you have diabetes for two main reasons. First, as we have seen, prolonged raised blood glucose levels can result in reduced sensation caused by nerve damage, and this is particularly common in the feet. This means that you may not feel pain from minor injuries such as cuts or grazes, blisters from a new pair of shoes or even an ingrown toenail – if you don't feel the pain of the nail growing into the flesh, the condition remains untreated. Likewise, if you don't feel the blister on the sole of your foot, you continue to walk on it so it quickly becomes worse and may develop into an ulcer. Second, diabetes increases your risk of narrowing of the arteries – the 'furring' up of the lining of the arteries caused by a build up of fatty deposits. This means blood flow to various parts of the body is restricted, making the skin more vulnerable to damage in the first place. In addition, because decreased blood flow prevents oxygen and nutrients needed for repair from reaching the tissues, the restricted blood flow slows down the healing process of any wound or injury that has occurred. Therefore a tiny cut under the toe, which would be no more than an irritation to someone without diabetes, could eventually develop into an ulcer in someone with diabetes.

Bob is 62 and has had type 2 diabetes for 17 years. He has always been very careful about examining his feet but he now has a foot infection that, although he is receiving treatment, is causing him some distress. 'I've lost a lot of feeling in my feet, so I know I might not feel any cuts or grazes, but I'm very careful to look them over at least a couple of times a week. What I didn't realize was just how bad my eyesight was getting. I wear glasses for driving but I can still see to read, so I didn't think I needed them for looking at my feet. I didn't notice anything until I took my sock off one night and found it was wet. I thought I might have cut myself and as I looked at my foot, I was mentally preparing myself to see it covered in blood, but actually it was almost worse – my heel was swollen and obviously infected. It was oozing pus which I could smell, a horrible sweet, sickly, rotten smell. And yet it didn't hurt! My wife rang the out-of-hours doctor and they sent a nurse round to clean and dress it. She said there was an ulcer developing, and she found a tiny stone embedded in my heel. She said it must have got into my shoe and, because of the nerve damage to my heel, I just didn't feel it. She was surprised I didn't see it, though, and suggested I have my eyes tested. She also said I should check my feet every day, which I shall do from now on. Ironically, even though I'm concerned about the infection in my foot, which is taking ages to heal, it turned out that the diabetes has started to cause some damage in my eyes, so that I need a different lens prescription and I really should be wearing glasses all the time. The optician says it's not too bad, but I do need to watch my blood glucose. And I'll make sure I wear glasses when I check my feet in future!'

Our feet are particularly vulnerable to injury, simply because we walk around on them all day and, if you have some loss of sensation as a result of diabetes, you may not notice the everyday problems that, for someone without diabetes, would be a minor irritation – an in-growing toenail, an abrasion or blister due to tight shoes, or like Bob, a stone in the shoe digging into your flesh. If you have diabetes you must be on constant watch for signs of nerve damage and of poor blood flow to the feet, because this can eventually lead to gangrene.

Gangrene

Gangrene is the death of tissue, most common in the legs and feet, caused by inadequate blood supply or bacterial infection of an open sore or ulcer. Anyone with poor circulation can develop gangrene, but it is more common in people with diabetes who have associated loss of circulation in the feet and toes.

One of the warning signs that blood flow is obstructed is sudden pain in the feet or legs together with a decrease in skin temperature. Unfortunately, if you have reduced sensation in your feet because of diabetic neuropathy, you're less likely to feel pain or to notice the change in temperature. Another sign is a change in skin colour of the affected area. Skin may appear pale at first, then become red and hot before turning purple and eventually black over a few days.

Treatment involves surgical removal of the gangrenous tissues and also living tissue from the surrounding area if it is infected. Antibiotics may be given to treat infection and, if possible, doctors will attempt to restore the blood supply. If an artery has become narrowed, even a tiny blood clot will be enough to obstruct blood flow. It may be possible to widen the artery using a technique called angioplasty, in which a balloon on the tip of a catheter or probe is passed into the artery and then inflated. Alternatively, the blockage may be surgically removed, or a femoral artery bypass graft carried out. This is where a section of vein from the same leg is grafted onto the artery so that blood can flow freely past the blocked section.

What to look out for:
Signs of poor circulation, including:

- Cold feet
- Red or purplish skin when your feet are hanging down, and a whitening of the skin when you lift your feet above the level of your heart

33

- Shiny, thin-looking skin
- Dry, flaky skin
- Loss of hair on the toes
- Pain in calves when walking
- Pain or throbbing at night or when at rest

Signs of nerve damage, including:

- Skin that feels hot to the touch
- Gradual loss of sensation in parts of the foot
- Muscle weakness in part of all of the foot (sometimes called drop foot)
- Numbness, tingling
- Pain or burning sensation
- Swelling

What you can do to keep your feet healthy

If you haven't already done so, you really must give up smoking – apart from the enormous health risks associated with smoking that you'll already be aware of, smoking does the same thing to your arteries (causing them to narrow and harden) that your diabetes is already doing; therefore, if you smoke, you're asking for double trouble!

- Keep close watch on your blood glucose – as we've seen, high blood glucose can damage the blood vessels.
- Check your feet daily for any signs of injury, including ingrown toenails and blisters. If you can't see your own feet properly, use a mirror or get someone else to do it for you.

Steps you can take to avoid foot injuries:

- Don't go barefoot, and always check for small stones or grit in shoes or other footwear before you put them on.
- Check the temperature of bathwater before you get in.
- Don't put your feet too close to the fire.
- Don't wear shoes that rub or are too tight – if necessary, go to a

specialist shoe shop where you can get shoes that are broad enough, deep enough and soft enough while still offering support for the foot. If the shoes feel too tight, don't hope they'll 'give' after you've worn them for a while – just don't buy them! Shoes that have laces, buckles or Velcro fastening are better than 'slip-ons' as they stop your feet from moving around in the shoe.

- Always wear socks with shoes or boots, but don't wear socks or tights that cramp your toes (which could cause ingrown toenails) or that are too tight (which could affect the circulation).
- Cut toenails frequently. Make sure you cut them straight across and not too short.
- If you have corns, calluses, verrucae or ingrown toenails, see a health professional such as a chiropodist or podiatrist rather than trying to attend to the problem yourself.
- Wash and dry your feet carefully every day. Moisturize dry skin, but not between the toes since this area is moist anyway and vulnerable to infections such as athlete's foot, which can cause the skin to crack and flake. If you do develop athlete's foot, see your doctor or treat it yourself with an anti-fungal cream from your pharmacy.
- Treat minor cuts, abrasions or blisters immediately. Wash with soap and water and use antibiotic cream. Don't pop blisters! If the wound doesn't seem to be healing, or if you're not sure how to treat it, seek medical advice.

All this talk of ulcers, gangrene and amputation is obviously quite scary, but while it's very important to keep your feet healthy and keep a close watch for any sign of problems, it should be borne in mind that foot problems – and many of the other problems mentioned in this chapter for that matter – are not inevitable if you have diabetes. The important thing is to control your condition as best you can in order to avoid or limit damage to the nerves and blood vessels that could lead to these complications.

5

The role of diet in treatment and prevention

Although there are many risk factors for type 2 diabetes that we can't change, such as our age, ethnicity and genetic make-up, we know that we can influence two of the biggest risk factors – weight and activity level. By making even minor adjustments to diet and lifestyle we can significantly reduce our risk of developing the disease. And if you've already been diagnosed or if you develop type 2 diabetes in the future, you can minimize the risks of diabetes-related complications. For this reason the 'first-line' treatment many doctors recommend is a combination of diet and exercise (see Chapters 5 and 6 for more on how exercise can help.) And you'll be pleased to hear that a diagnosis of diabetes doesn't necessarily mean that you'll have to follow a special diet or give up chocolate. In fact, a recent Italian study suggested that chocolate might actually be good for people with diabetes. The study found that eating 100 grams of dark chocolate each day for 15 days lowered blood pressure and improved the body's ability to metabolize sugar. But a word of caution – Diabetes UK said the study was interesting and agreed that people with diabetes can eat dark chocolate like everyone else in moderation. However, they pointed out that the study was a very small one (it involved just 15 people) and they continue to recommend a balanced diet that is low in fat, salt and sugar and that includes starchy carbohydrates and plenty of fruit and vegetables, combined with regular exercise.

There is no special diet for people with diabetes – the healthy diet for people with diabetes is the healthy diet recommended for everyone. If you're overweight, however, or if you already have health problems such as high blood pressure or high cholesterol, you may need to pay more attention to your diet for a while to get these things under control.

Does your diet need attention?

Even if you're not overweight, you can still benefit from overhauling your diet. If you can honestly say that you drink plenty of water, eat five portions of fruit and vegetables a day, that your diet is low in salt, sugar and saturated fat and high in starchy carbohydrates, and that you always have your oily fish quota, then you can skip this section and go straight on to reading about exercise.

Still here? Thought so. Most of us know at least a little about what we should be eating and many of us make real efforts to keep our diets healthy, but the reality is, with the stresses and strains of everyday life, the speed with which we often need to shop and cook and eat, the diets of most of the population range from less than perfect to seriously unhealthy. When we talk about a western diet being unhealthy, we usually mean a diet that's high in fats, sugar and processed foods, although it may also be unhealthy in other ways. If we eat too much fat and sugar, we gain weight. If we gain weight, we put a strain on the body's systems and this ultimately leads to disease. As we have already seen, being overweight is the single biggest risk factor for type 2 diabetes and obesity itself is said to be reaching 'epidemic' proportions in the UK, where 22 per cent of adults are now classified as obese, and in the USA, where the number of adults who are overweight or obese is around 33 per cent. But even if you are not overweight, there are probably ways in which your diet could be improved in order to maintain a healthy weight and to keep your blood glucose under control.

What is a healthy weight?

You'll find numerous magazine articles with charts to help you calculate your 'ideal weight', but rather than aiming for a 'goal weight', what you should be looking at is getting your weight down to within a healthy range, and that may be several pounds either side of what the charts tell you. The range that's healthy for you will depend on many factors, including your age, sex and build. The body mass index (BMI) is a formula that uses weight and height to estimate body fat and gauge the potential health risks caused by excess weight. According to the World Health Organization, a BMI of between 18 and 25 is healthy, whereas a BMI of between 25 and 30 would suggest you are overweight. If your BMI is more than 30, you would be classified as obese. (See page 15) for how to calculate your BMI.)

The BMI gives a fairly good guide but it has its limitations and is only one factor in determining an individual's health risk. BMI does not take into account lean body mass or body frame, for example, so a six foot tall, large-framed footballer may well have a BMI that suggests overweight or even obesity. But muscle tissue is heavier than fat, and so a muscular body that, on paper, seems heavy for that person's height may in fact be super-fit and healthy. Recently, experts have suggested that a person's shape and in particular, the waist measurement, may be a better indication of risk when it comes to diseases such as diabetes and cardiovascular diseases. A waist measurement of more than 40 inches (102 centimetres) for men and more than 35 inches (88 centimetres) for women is regarded as 'abdominal obesity', and indicates a need to take action.

The chances are you'll know deep down whether you need to lose weight or not. If you're not sure, take your clothes off, stand in front of the mirror and take a candid look – do you see wobbly bits? Exercise will help tone flabby flesh, but if it's fat flabby flesh, you need to look at your diet.

If you are overweight, your risk of developing type 2 diabetes is at least double that of someone who is not. If you are classified as obese, that risk is up to 10 times greater. And if you're seriously obese – if your BMI is more than 35 – your risk is up to 80 times greater than that of someone with a healthy BMI of less then 22. The vast majority of people with type 2 diabetes are overweight when diagnosed, many of them significantly so. But even losing small amounts of weight can help lower blood glucose, and a weight loss of around 10 per cent will be enough to considerably reduce the risk of developing complications such as heart disease and stroke.

Don't aim to lose too much too quickly – research has shown that rapid weight loss simply leads to equally rapid weight gain. Think less about the weight you want to get to and more about changing your eating habits for good – if you 'go on a diet', the implication is that you will adopt a particular way of eating for a certain period of time, and when that period of time is over or the 'goal' weight reached, you will 'come off' the diet and return to your original eating habits. This may work temporarily, but has two main flaws. First, 'going on a diet' often involves depriving yourself of foods you enjoy. If you feel deprived, you're more likely to cave in one day and gobble up a whole chocolate cake or a double cheeseburger with mayonnaise and a large portion of fries. Second, it was your original eating habits that led to the weight gain in the first place, so if you return to the same pattern of eating, chances are you'll put back on all that you lost. 'Crash' or fast weight loss diets don't work for the same reasons but also because, if we suddenly start taking in only very small amounts of food, our bodies go on 'starvation alert', conserving as much energy as possible from the small amount of nutrients available. So if, for example, you ate only 800 calories a day while dieting, if you then started eating 1,500 calories a day (many people would lose weight on 1,500 calories) you would actually start to gain weight again because your body has become used to running effectively on less fuel, so the surplus calories will be stored as fat.

If, on the other hand, you content yourself with a slow but steady weight loss and you don't worry too much if you only lose half a pound two weeks running, you're more likely to find your new way of eating is sustainable for much longer, especially if you incorporate a little gentle daily exercise to help things along. Then, when you eventually reach a healthy weight, you can very gradually increase the amount you eat while sticking to the same healthy eating principles, so that you maintain your new weight without difficulty.

Keep a food diary

Extra weight often creeps on gradually. In your teens and twenties, you may be sylph-like, full of energy and able to wear anything you like. But as life wears on, you have kids, you give up badminton, you watch more television, you take to having a few beers after work or a couple of glasses of wine with dinner and gradually, over time, you become twice the man or woman you used to be. The best way to identify the problems with your diet is to keep a food diary for a week or two. Make sure you write down every tiny morsel that passes your lips. Even if you're not overweight, it's easy to be unaware of every single thing that goes into your mouth – how often do you eat up the crusts from the kids' toast in the morning or that last roast potato in the pan without even noticing? And don't forget drinks – an extra cappuccino or glass of fruit juice on a daily basis can make quite a difference over a week.

Keeping a food diary requires commitment, so don't make it too hard for yourself at first: just note down what you consumed and when, especially if it's not a normal mealtime. This will help you to identify times when you may be eating because of boredom rather than because you're hungry. It may also show you specific times when you're more likely to eat an unhealthy snack because it's convenient. If you can identify bad eating habits, you'll be able to change them more easily. If, for example, you frequently grab a high-fat sandwich or a couple of croissants on the way to work because you didn't have time for breakfast, or you end up eating a burger or fried chicken for lunch because that's all they have in the work canteen, you can see that setting your alarm for half an hour earlier would allow you time to make a healthy sandwich for lunch and to eat some muesli and yoghurt before you leave the house. Even if you made no other changes, just changing that one daily habit would help you lose weight and establish more healthy eating.

What is healthy eating?

We all know we're supposed to eat a balanced diet, but what exactly does that mean? All foods fall into certain groups and, in order to eat a balanced diet, we need foods from each of those groups, but in varying quantities. In general, there is no one food that you can't eat, even if you have diabetes, but the amount you eat is important, especially when it comes to foods that are high in fat or sugar (or both). It is a myth that people with diabetes can't eat sugar, but sugary foods should make up only a very small amount of your total daily food intake as should foods that are high in fat. The Diabetes Food Pyramid, devised by the American Diabetes Association, is a simple way of visualising this. At the bottom is the carbohydrate group: bread, cereal, rice, pasta and potatoes. Starchy carbohydrates provide the most energy, and should make up the bulk of your diet. Depending on your height and weight, you should eat six to eleven servings from this group daily. One slice of bread or a small bowl of cereal counts as a serving.

The fruit and vegetable groups come next. These are good sources of many vitamins and minerals, and they help to boost the immune system. Aim for at least three to five servings of vegetables each day and two to four servings of fruit – but bear in mind that the natural sugars in fruit can raise your blood glucose levels significantly, so treat fruit more cautiously than vegetables. One serving of fruit is one item such as an apple or orange or a handful of berries. A small glass of fruit juice also counts as a portion of fruit, but if you have or are at risk of diabetes, it's best to stick to whole fruit if possible – the sugar (fructose, or fruit sugar) in fruit juice is concentrated and can send your blood glucose soaring. One large carrot or a medium portion of salad or greens counts as one serving of vegetables.

You need smaller amounts from the next two groups, which are the milk and yoghurt group and the meat, fish and cheese group. Milk and yoghurt, along with cheese, provide calcium for healthy bones and some protein. The biggest sources of protein are meat and poultry, fish, eggs, nuts, and pulses such as lentils and beans. Eat two to three servings a day from each of these two groups. A serving would be an egg or four ounces of cooked lean meat or fish or one small portion of lentils.

The smallest section at the top of the pyramid is that from which we should eat sparingly. This includes sugar, fats and oils. Sweets, cakes, biscuits and preserves have little nutritional value, are high in calories and will increase your blood glucose sharply, so they really should be kept for a once-in-a-while treat. Fats are slightly more complicated.

Fats and oils

Everyone needs to consume a certain amount of fat, but it's the type of fat that we eat that has a major bearing on our health, with high cholesterol levels increasing the risk of several diseases, including type 2 diabetes, heart disease and stroke.

Cholesterol

Cholesterol is essential to the body and plays an important role in building cell membranes and in the manufacture of certain hormones. The body manufactures a certain amount of its own cholesterol and the rest comes from dietary sources. After we've eaten a meal, the liver takes up cholesterol and triglycerides from the blood and packages them into tiny spheres called lipoproteins. The lipoproteins, a combination of cholesterol, triglycerides and certain proteins, are transported in the bloodstream to the cells of the body, where the various components are extracted as required.

41

There are two types of cholesterol; 'bad' cholesterol, which is associated with low-density lipoprotein (LDL) and 'good' cholesterol, which is associated with high-density lipoprotein (HDL). Most cholesterol in the blood comes from LDL, and when doctors refer to high cholesterol levels, they are usually referring to LDL. If you have high LDL cholesterol levels, the LDL tends to stick to the lining of the arteries, causing atheroscleroris and a build-up of plaque. This results in narrowed arteries, which can lead to heart attack, stroke and neuropathy.

The 'good' cholesterol comes from HDL, but this represents only a small proportion of blood cholesterol. There is now considerable evidence that higher levels of HDL are associated with a lower risk of cardiovascular disease, while low HDL levels are associated with increased risk. Although we do not know for sure why HDL appears to reduce the risk, there is some evidence to suggest that HDL seems to scour the walls of the blood vessels, cleaning out the excess cholesterol and then carrying it back to the liver for further processing.

There are several factors associated with increased levels of LDL cholesterol in your blood, and some of these, such as age, sex and family history, cannot be altered. However, there are other factors you can influence, such as giving up smoking (see page 24), increasing the amount of exercise in your daily routine (see Chapter 6) and changing your diet. Although diet is only responsible for a relatively small amount of cholesterol in the body – most is produced by the liver – a diet high in saturated fats can actually cause the liver to produce more LDL cholesterol. Exactly how much diet influences cholesterol levels varies from person to person. Some people who eat high-fat diets have high cholesterol levels, whereas others manage to get away with normal or even low cholesterol levels. Likewise, some people may struggle to keep their cholesterol levels under control, even when sticking to relatively low-fat diets. In most cases, however, switching to a low-fat diet will reduce cholesterol levels and help achieve or maintain a healthy weight.

The worse culprits for increasing LDL cholesterol are saturated fats – those found in animal fats such as meat, lard and dairy products. Unsaturated fats – those that come mainly from plant sources or fish – are much healthier and often contain HDL ('good') cholesterol. Unsaturated fats may be monounsaturated – sources include avocados, almonds, hazelnuts, and peanut, rapeseed and olive oils – or polyunsaturated, which can be found in soya, sunflower and corn oils, walnuts, seeds, wheatgerm, and fish oils. Studies show that polyunsaturates and, to a lesser extent, monounsaturates can help lower blood cholesterol levels, thus helping to protect the heart and reduce the risk of cardiovascular disease.

There are some types of fatty acids that cannot be made within the body but that are vital for health. These are called essential fatty acids – 'essential' because we need to take them in, in the form of food, on a regular basis, so they are an essential part of our diet. Essential fatty acids are needed for the formation of cell walls, and so are vital for growth and repair of tissues. They are also necessary for a variety of other functions, including skin repair, brain function and immune system function. There are two types of essential fatty acids, omega-3 and omega-6. Good sources of omega-3 fatty acids include soya bean and rapeseed oils, as well as fish, especially oily varieties such as sardines, herring, mackerel, trout and salmon. We need around 1–2 grams a day, and this can be provided by a 100 gram portion of herring, or a handful of walnuts. Omega-6 is found in many vegetable oils, especially sunflower, olive and corn oil. The daily requirement is about 4 g a day, which is equal to two teaspoons of sunflower oil or a handful of almonds or walnuts.

Essential fatty acids should not be confused with trans fatty acids. Trans fatty acids, like saturated fats, also increase cholesterol levels and are therefore detrimental to heart health. Ironically, trans fatty acids are the result of manufacturers trying to make products more healthy. When the dangers associated with saturated fats were identified, the food industry wanted to switch to using unsaturated fatty acids. The trouble was that unsaturated fatty acids turn rancid fairly quickly, so manufacturers began to 'hydrogenate' them, a process that forms a more solid and longer-lasting form of vegetable oil called 'partially hydrogenated' oil. Unfortunately, a side effect of the process of hydrogenation is the formation of another type of fatty acid – trans fatty acid. So when manufacturers began to use partially hydrogenated vegetable oils instead of saturated fats in their processed foods, they began adding large amounts of trans fatty acids. Fortunately, it's fairly easy to identify foods that contain large amounts of trans fatty acids: solid magarines (the harder the margarine, the higher it is in trans fatty acids), high-fat bakery products such as cakes, biscuits and doughnuts, fried goods such as chips and potato crisps and anything that says 'partially hydrogenated vegetable oils' on the ingredients label – usually manufactured and processed foods.

Treating type 2 diabetes with diet

If you've already been diagnosed, you should be receiving information and support from a dietician as part of your treatment plan. Although the dietary rules for treating diabetes are very similar to those for avoiding or delaying its development, it's important to devise a diet plan that suits your individual needs, taking into account things like lifestyle and cultural preferences as well as any specific health or weight issues. In general, a diet for treating diabetes aims to:

- Achieve normal or near-normal blood glucose levels (i.e. 4–7 mmol/l)
- Keep blood glucose levels under control
- Control blood pressure
- Protect the heart and keep it healthy by controlling cholesterol levels
- Achieve a reasonable, sustainable weight
- Manage or prevent complications of diabetes
- Keep you fit and healthy

If your health warrants an immediate drastic change in diet – for example, if you are very overweight and your health-care team considers you to be seriously at risk of heart problems or stroke, you'll probably be given very detailed information of what you should be eating and how much. But in many cases, the advice will be more general and will be based around changing your diet to take in basic healthy eating principles such as reducing sugar, fat and salt intake, increasing the amount of fruit and vegetables you eat, and so on. It may seem daunting to have to change the way you eat, but believe it or not, these changes can be achieved fairly easily. Here are a few simple tips to help you plan your new diet.

- Plan regular meals around high-fibre, starchy foods.
- Eating regularly helps to keep your blood glucose levels stable, as

44

does having starchy carbohydrates, which also provide energy, as the main part of your meal.

- Have a smaller amount of protein and plenty of vegetables or salad.
- Good sources of starchy carbohydrates include: potatoes, yams, rice, pasta, noodles, plantain, chapatis, bread and cereal. Choose wholemeal or wholegrain varieties where possible because these are high in fibre and help prevent constipation.
- Other fibre-rich foods include fruit, vegetables and pulses. Many of these contain soluble fibre, which can reduce absorption of cholesterol into the bloodstream and may reduce the risk of harmful blood clots. Other sources of soluble fibre include oats, barley, brown rice and some seeds.

Reduce your sugar intake

The good news is that you don't have to give up sugar completely! However, sugar contains 'empty' calories – units of energy that contain few nutrients and will therefore be stored by the body as fat – so you need to keep a close eye on sugar consumption. It's worth bearing in mind that many foods contain hidden sugars. Baked beans, for example, may contain some sugar, though it's unlikely to be enough to have any real effect on your blood glucose levels. Fruit drinks, squashes and fizzy drinks can be very high in sugar and can send your blood glucose soaring, so choose sugar-free or diet alternatives. You don't have to deny yourself sugary foods such as cakes, biscuits or desserts for ever more, but keep them for an occasional treat. Minimize any adverse effect on your blood glucose by having your treat as part of your regular carbohydrate-based, high-fibre meal and sticking to tiny portions.

Cut down on fat

Although fat doesn't directly affect your blood glucose, it's important in weight control and, if you're overweight, reducing your intake will help you lose weight and reduce your risk of heart disease. Try to reduce the total amount of fat in your diet, especially saturated fat (see the section on fats and oils, page 41). Choose low-fat options where possible, but read the labels – some low fat products may not necessarily be 'healthy' if they're high in sugar or salt.

- Use skimmed or semi-skimmed milk.
- Use an olive oil-based or other low-fat spread instead of butter or hard margarine.
- Choose lower-fat cheeses such as Edam, Brie or half-fat cheddar (but don't overdo the cheese!).
- Poach, grill or bake rather than fry. When stir-frying, use an olive oil spray or brush the oil on with a pastry brush.
- Choose fat-free salad dressings.
- Low-fat yoghurt or fromage frais makes a good alternative to cream or ice cream.
- Have larger portions of vegetables or salad and smaller portions of meat.
- Choose lower fat meats and trim off visible fat. Remove skin from chicken.
- Cut right down on fatty processed meat products such as sausages and burgers.

Reduce your salt intake

A high intake of salt and salty foods can lead to high blood pressure and increase your risk of heart disease and stroke. In the UK the average adult's daily consumption of salt is around 9 grams. The Government recommends this be reduced to 6 grams. Reducing the amount of salt you use is about re-educating your taste buds. If you're used to a lot of salt in your diet, there's no point in pretending it'll be easy to cut your intake drastically, but it may be easier in the long run than cutting down gradually. Try this for a couple of weeks: cut out all salty foods such as crisps, salted nuts, stock cubes and processed foods such as soups, pizzas and ready meals, don't use salt at the table and stop adding it to cooking. It'll be strange at first, but stick with it. Try using more garlic and other herbs and spices to add flavour. After two or three weeks, your taste receptors will be far more sensitive and you'll find salty foods quite unpleasant.

Most of the salt in our diets comes from processed foods rather than from salt added at the cooking or serving stage. Therefore, in order to keep an eye on your intake, you really need to read the labels. But these can be confusing. A recent study found that many people thought that sodium and salt were the same thing. In fact, to find the salt content of a product, you need to multiply the amount of sodium by 2.5. As a rough guide, a food that contains 0.5 grams of sodium per 100 grams is considered a high-salt food, whereas 0.1 grams per 100 grams is fine.

Watch your alcohol consumption

Although the odd drink won't hurt you, alcohol is fairly high in calories and, like sugar, has little nutritional value. Some studies show that moderate alcohol consumption may actually reduce the risk of type 2 diabetes, and there is evidence to suggest that moderate drinkers are less at risk of heart disease than teetotallers. However, the key is moderate consumption – drinking too much can lead to excess weight and has an adverse affect on general health. The best advice is to stick to the Government's recommended safe limits (i.e. no more than two units a day for women and three for men). You should also have at least two alcohol-free days a week. If you have diabetes, it's best not to drink alcohol on an empty stomach because this can cause a sudden fall in blood glucose levels.

More fruit and vegetables

You're probably sick of hearing it by now, but apart from giving up smoking and reducing your intake of saturated fats, eating more fruit and veg is probably the single most beneficial change you can make to your lifestyle in terms of health. Try for a couple of pieces of fruit a day and at least three portions of vegetables. Not only will these healthy foods fill you up and provide essential fibre, they are also an excellent source of vitamins and antioxidants, and they will help to protect you against a number of diseases, including several types of cancer.

If you loathe lettuce or can't bear broccoli, think about sneaky ways of increasing your intake. Try making vegetable soups or adding extra vegetables to casseroles and stews. Chargrilled Mediterranean vegetables go well with fish or on a thin-crust pizza, or you could throw a handful of mushrooms or sweetcorn into an omelette, pile coleslaw into a jacket potato or have baked beans or tomatoes on toast for breakfast. If you think salads are boring, try mixing finely chopped mixed peppers, cucumber, tomato and red onion. Add a few capers, chopped olives and a fat-free dressing of your choice – delicious! All these ideas help to add to your daily vegetable count. Most people have less trouble eating enough fruit, but if this is a problem for you, don't forget that a glass of fruit juice counts as a portion (watch your blood-glucose levels, though) as does dried fruit such as prunes or apricots. Try adding chopped fruit to yoghurt or fromage frais, or making a sugar-free fruit salad for dessert.

And if you still need convincing, next time you go to the supermarket, look at the wonderful displays of colourful fresh fruit and vegetables, remember the old saying, 'you are what you eat', and then just picture yourself shining with health like a rosy apple instead of glistening with fat like a sweaty jam doughnut!

Glycaemic index

The glycaemic index (GI) is a way of measuring how quickly carbohydrate-containing foods raise blood glucose levels after being eaten. Foods are given a GI of 1–100 depending on how quickly they are metabolized. The GI compares the body's response to the carbohydrate in a particular food with its reaction to pure glucose, which is given the value of 100. So, for example, if a food raises blood glucose only half as much as pure glucose, that food is given a GI of 50. The portion size tested is the amount that contains 50 grams of carbohydrate. This shows us that foods that contain the same amount of carbohydrate do not raise blood glucose levels at the same rate, as scientists previously thought. We now know, for example, that 30 grams of carbohydrate as bread does not have the same effect as 30 grams of carbohydrate as pasta.

The GI of a food depends on several factors, including the form of carbohydrate it contains, the amount and form of fibre it contains, how it has been cooked or processed and whether other substances such as fats or protein are present. Foods with a GI of less than 55 are broken down more slowly and are considered to be 'low', whereas a food with a GI of more than 70 is considered 'high' as it will be converted into glucose much more quickly. Foods with a GI of between 55 and 70 are considered 'moderate'. Basically, the higher the GI, the quicker the jump in blood glucose, while foods with a lower GI will allow blood glucose to rise more slowly.

Why choose a low GI diet?

A low GI diet is not the perfect solution that some diet books suggest, but it may help prevent and control type 2 diabetes, and some people may find it helps them to lose weight. Critics point out that the way foods are measured – one food at a time and in portion sizes that contain the same amount of carbohydrate – does not reflect how we really eat, which tends to be several foods together and in varying quantities. Another criticism is that some low GI foods (such as ice cream or peanuts) contain large amount of fats or sugar and could result in weight gain. Overall, though, many experts agree that a low GI diet can certainly have benefits if used sensibly.

Generally speaking, foods with a lower GI make you feel full for longer periods of time, so you tend to eat less, thus helping you to lose weight. Slow-acting carbohydrates also reduce the peaks in blood glucose that often follow a meal, and keeping blood glucose levels down is one of the most important factors in reducing the risk of type 2 diabetes. Research has shown that changing to a low GI diet can reduce insulin resistance and the risk of heart disease and lower levels of 'bad' (LDL) cholesterol.

How do you eat a low GI diet?

The GI only tells us how quickly a food raises blood glucose when eaten alone. However, in practice, we may eat bread with cheese, fish with chips, meat with potatoes and so on. So it's not as simple as cutting out high GI foods and eating more low GI foods – chocolate is low, for example, as are sausages and potato crisps, and eating too much of these foods is likely to lead to weight gain and to contribute to cardiovascular problems. Instead, just as you would with any pattern of healthy eating, try to think about the overall balance of your meals. Include plenty of starchy foods, plenty of vegetables and fruit, plus foods that are low in fat, sugar and salt. If you eat low GI foods along with those that are moderate or high, you can lower the overall GI of your meal, so include at least one low GI food with each meal, and make low GI foods the main component of at least two meals a day.

If you decide you want to follow a low GI diet, you may be able to get some advice from your diabetes health-care team on what foods to eat. Generally speaking, good foods to include are low-fat, high-fibre foods that have undergone little processing. For example, mixed or multigrain breads that contain whole grains tend to have a lower GI than 'wholewheat' or 'wholemeal' breads – although the whole grain may have been used in wholemeal breads, it will have been ground up instead of left whole. This means the body can break it down more quickly than whole grains. The fibrous coat around beans and lentils also slows down absorption, ranking them lower on the GI scale. Brown rice is higher in fibre than white rice and is digested more slowly, so it also has a lower GI.

Low GI foods include:

- Legumes (lentils, beans, chick peas) and legume products such as baked beans, hummus, lentil soup and dhal
- Wholegrain breads
- Cereals, especially porridge, most muesli and some bran-based breakfast cereals
- Nuts
- Chapatis
- Pasta
- Sweet potato and yam
- Most vegetables and fruits
- Chocolate – but beware! It's also high in fat and sugar

Foods with a medium GI include:

- Wholemeal bread
- Brown or basmati rice
- Boiled potatoes
- Honey and jam
- Couscous
- Tinned fruit
- Sultanas and raisins

High GI foods include:

- Glucose
- White bread, French bread
- White rice
- Bagels
- Crumpets
- Mashed potato
- Cornflakes

Low GI menu ideas:

- Breakfast – porridge, muesli or a bran-based cereal, plus a few strawberries
- Lunch – jacket potato with baked beans, lentil soup with a wholegrain roll, or dhal with a chapati
- Dinner – aim for pasta-based meals with low-fat sauces, or base meals around basmati rice, noodles, sweet potato or pearl barley. Try to include more beans and pulses
- Snacks – fruit, raw vegetables, low-fat yoghurt (but watch the sugar content of fruit yoghurts)

If you're keen on trying to follow a healthy eating plan based on the glycaemic index, see *The Glycaemic Factor: How to balance your blood sugar* by Theresa Cheung (Sheldon Press, 2005), or see Further reading on page 113.

6

The role of exercise in treatment and prevention

In the Western world of the twenty-first century, our lives have become more and more sedentary. We drive to work, we sit at a computer all day, we send out for lunch and drive home again for an evening in front of the television. The remote control means we don't even have to get up to change the channel. No wonder so many of us are unfit and overweight. And no wonder the idea of vigorous exercise sends us scurrying for the security of a comfy armchair and a bar of chocolate!

All of us, no matter how inactive, no matter how long it is since we last made an effort to exercise, can incorporate at least a little extra movement into our daily routine. You should of course check with your doctor before undertaking any new physical activity, especially if you are seriously overweight, pregnant or elderly or if you already have other health problems.

The benefits of exercise

Probably the most obvious benefit of becoming more physically active is that it helps those who need to lose weight do so more quickly. It also helps to lower and control blood glucose levels. Exercise causes your body to burn more calories and to use insulin more efficiently than if you were sitting watching television. It causes blood to be pumped around the body faster, strengthening your heart and the other muscles you use for movement; it also burns fat and cholesterol and improves your muscle tone. You'll feel better and look trimmer, and the effect on your blood glucose will help prevent type 2 diabetes from developing, or at the very least delay its onset. After half an hour of moderate exercise, most people's blood glucose levels drop by 20–25 per cent. This is because during and after exercise, the body produces less glucose, uses glucose more easily and develops new insulin receptors on the cell membranes. And it's not just the body that improves as you gradually increase your levels of activity and movement. Exercise also has a beneficial affect on the mind, helping to combat depression by causing the brain to release certain 'happy chemicals' – hormones that lift mood – into the bloodstream. It also helps to reduce stress, improve memory and boost confidence and self-image.

But I hate exercise . . .

If you haven't exercised since you were at school, you're probably terrified of exposing all that flesh and running around making everything bounce. But don't worry. You don't have to go to the gym or buy a step machine or even watch a video of some skinny celebrity prancing around in a pink leotard. We are talking about a change of lifestyle here, not a burst of strenuous exercise that'll make you ache all over and put you off for ever. You need to develop a programme of activity that suits who you are and fits in with your daily routine, something that you know you can keep up and hopefully improve on as your fitness increases. Ideally, it should be based around something you enjoy doing, or can at least tolerate. If you really can't bear the thought of a structured exercise programme, start by simply incorporating more activity into your daily routine. Once you start to feel fitter and less sluggish, you may find you're more willing to consider other forms of exercise.

In the meantime, think about your daily routine. Do you go out to work or is your daily work centred around the home? Could you walk part of the way to work? Park the car a little further from the office? Get off the bus or train one stop earlier? If that's impossible, when you get to work, could you take the stairs instead of the lift? Could you go for a walk at lunchtime? If you just took a 25-minute walk during your lunchbreak, you'll have clocked up more than two hours of exercise at the end of the working week. If you're at home with the kids, do you need to drive them to school or nursery? Perhaps they'd benefit from the extra exercise, too. You could use the time to chat about school or help them learn their alphabet or nine times table. If you run your business from home, particularly if it involves lots of time sitting at your desk, it can be very difficult to make yourself move. But maybe you could make a point of taking a walk at lunchtime. Many self-employed people say they 'don't have time' for lunch breaks, but research has shown that taking regular breaks from your daily work actually improves efficiency and output.

Finding what's right for you

The best type of exercise, whether you have diabetes or not, is aerobic or cardiovascular exercise – low-intensity, long-duration activity that increases the heart rate, makes you sweat and works the circulatory system. Examples are walking, swimming and cycling. If you haven't exercised for years, you'll need to build up slowly. For some people, joining a gym is the answer, but many who do so give up in the first few months, either because they have trouble finding the time to actually go to the gym, or because they find it boring or intimidating. It can also be expensive. But there are plenty of other ways you can exercise. Think about the sort of person you are and the things you enjoy doing. Do you like the great outdoors or are you more of an indoor person? Are you sociable and outgoing or are you happier in your own company or with a partner or close friend? Could you persuade someone to exercise with you, or would you be more comfortable alone? What about your children or grandchildren? Could you combine spending quality time with the kids with an activity that would help you to get fit? Thinking about your work, hobbies, interests, family and friends may give you some ideas as to how to devise the most appropriate programme of exercise. As your fitness increases, you may find you have the appetite for activities you wouldn't have previously considered. You can also start to increase the length of your exercise session, building up to an hour or so if possible. This is especially important in a weight-loss programme because the body starts to burn fat as fuel only after about 30–40 minutes of sustained aerobic activity.

Five golden rules

1. Any exercise is better than none. If all you can manage is 15 minutes extra housework or gardening a day, go for it, and rejoice in your shiny clean house, your neat and tidy garden and your improving health.
2. Exercise regularly – 20 minutes a day is better than a weekly two-

hour workout because not only do the calorie-burning effects last for some time after you stop exercising, but after several months of regular exercise, you'll also find your metabolism has actually changed, burning more calories all the time.

3. Be realistic about what you can achieve – if you set yourself too high a target, your exercise plan is doomed to fail. Start gradually, but be committed – you can always move on to more challenging workouts later, if you wish.

4. If you're using insulin or any other diabetes medication, test your blood glucose before, during and after exercising, and drink plenty of water!

5. Avoid injury – it's important to do five minutes or so of warm-up or stretching exercises, particularly for the legs. Diabetes can cause the nerve endings in your legs and feet to become less sensitive and so you may not feel pain in the ligaments that connect muscles to bones. This can result in torn ligaments or even broken bones. You should take special care of your feet because injury is more likely while exercising. Wear comfortable, well-fitting training shoes and be extra vigilant when checking for cuts, grazes and blisters. If you do hurt your feet, switch to a non-weight-bearing exercise such as swimming until the wound is completely healed.

Don't get bored

While it's important to exercise every day (or most days, at least), it's equally important to vary the type of exercise you do to avoid boredom setting in. Try to do at least two or three different things each week. Here are some activity ideas for you to think about.

- *Walking* – you can do it alone, with your partner, your children, a walkers' group or just your dog. You can go for a five-mile hike or a trot around the block. If you need to start very gradually, just get yourself walking around the house or garden a little more. You'll soon notice you're able to go further. Invest in a pedometer, an inexpensive device that clips onto your belt or waistband and measures the number of steps you take. It's a great motivational tool and will encourage you to do that little bit extra each day.

- *Take up golf* – it may seem like sport for the lazy, but walking around the course can burn up quite a few calories. The average golf course is three or four miles long, and if you carry or pull your clubs around with you as well, that's quite a workout. If you've never played before, it would be worth taking a few lessons – although injuries are rare, strains and sprains do sometimes occur in golfers who haven't learned how to move their bodies properly while perfecting their swing.
- *Swimming* – particularly good exercise if you're overweight, have back problems or are pregnant. Swimming is an excellent non-weight-bearing exercise. The water supports you, making injury less likely, and you can build up from a width or two of the pool to 20 or 30 lengths.
- *Cycling* – another great weight-bearing aerobic exercise and a cheap form of transport. Maybe a twice-weekly cycle ride as an alternative daily way of getting to work?

If you're not up to these types of exercise yet, think about other fun ways of increasing your activity levels. Take the kids to the park with a football, Frisbee or kite. Put some loud music on and dance around your kitchen while you're waiting for the dinner to cook, or offer to cut your neighbour's lawn as well as your own. Even if you have seriously reduced mobility as a result of age, weight or illness, you can still perform some stretching or muscle-strengthening exercises while sitting in a chair, perhaps to music to make it a little more interesting. Talk to your doctor or health practitioner about devising a suitable set of movements.

Exercise and blood glucose

Exercise draws on the body's reserves of glucose that are stored in your muscles and liver. As your body rebuilds its reserves, it takes glucose from your blood, thereby reducing your blood glucose level. This effect can last for several hours after the activity. The most effective time to exercise is when your blood glucose is at its highest which, for many people, is first thing in the morning. Starting your day with a 30-minute walk can help to keep your blood glucose low for much of the day, so it really is a good time to exercise. Fitness experts also recommend morning exercise because this is often the time of day when there are fewer demands on your time from family or work responsibilities.

If your diabetes is treated with insulin or some other medications, you need to check your blood glucose often (see Chapter 7), especially when you first begin to exercise. Make sure that your pre-exercise blood glucose isn't low. If it is, eat a starchy snack before you start, and test again to make sure it doesn't drop too low during and after exercise.

Tips to avoid low blood glucose levels while exercising

- Check your blood glucose levels twice before exercising, once about 30 minutes beforehand and then again right before you start. This will show you whether your blood glucose level is stable, rising or falling. For most people, a safe pre-exercise blood glucose range is around 5–9 mmol/l. If your blood glucose level is under 5 mmol/l, eat a carbohydrate-containing snack to avoid having low blood glucose (hypoglycaemia – often referred to as 'a hypo') while you exercise.

- Check your blood glucose again during exercise. This is especially important when you're trying a new activity or if you're increasing the intensity or duration of your exercise regime. If levels start to fall too low, have a snack. If you start to experience symptoms of hypoglycaemia, stop immediately and eat something with a fast-acting source of glucose, such as fruit juice or a few raisins.

- Check your blood glucose at least twice after exercise. The more strenuous the activity, the longer your blood glucose will be affected afterwards. Hypoglycaemia can occur hours after exercise, so you need to check your blood glucose levels quite frequently, at least until you get a clear picture of how your body reacts to exercise.

Stick with it – don't be discouraged if exercise causes significant changes in your blood glucose that interfere with your normal management routine. Eventually you'll notice a pattern and you'll be able to make changes to your meals and medications accordingly.

Although it may seem like a contradiction, in some circumstances physical activity can actually cause blood glucose levels to rise. This may occur if you already have a high blood glucose level (13 mmol/l or above). Having high blood glucose levels before exercise means there may not be enough insulin present in the body. When this happens, exercise stimulates the secretion of counter-regulatory hormones, which causes blood glucose to rise even further. So if your test shows a high reading before exercise, delay the session until your levels come down.

7

Treatment and testing

As we've seen, diet and exercise form the basis of treatment for type 2 diabetes. However, in around 25 per cent of those with type 2, the body does not produce enough insulin so lifestyle changes alone will not be enough to control blood glucose. In this case your doctor will prescribe diabetes pills or insulin, although you'll still be advised to follow a healthy diet and programme of exercise as well.

You may find that, while diet and exercise alone were enough to keep your blood glucose levels under control when you were first diagnosed, this may change over time. Diabetes is a progressive disease, so you may need to start taking diabetes pills, increase the dose or take more than one type of tablet; if your body stops producing insulin altogether, you may need to move on to insulin injections. In the UK, everyone whose diabetes is treated with insulin or diabetes tablets is exempt from prescription charges. And if your health-care team recommends that you test your blood glucose regularly (see page 70), you should be able to get testing equipment such as blood glucose monitoring meters or urine testing strips on prescription.

How do diabetes tablets work?

The many types of diabetes tablets work in different ways, and your doctor will decide which is the most suitable for you by taking various factors into account, including your age and weight and your heart, kidney and liver function. You may need to try several different tablets or combinations of tablets before you find the treatment best suited to you.

The main ways in which oral medication for diabetes works are by:

- Helping to reduce blood glucose levels
- Helping insulin to work more efficiently in the cells
- Boosting production of insulin in the pancreas
- Slowing absorption of glucose from the gut

What are the different types of diabetes tablets?

The five main types of diabetes tablets are listed below, including their generic (non-brand) names. Your doctor may prescribe the generic drug or may use a drug's brand name.

- Sulphonylureas, including chlorpropamide, glibenclamide, gliclazide, glimepiride, glipzide, gliquidine and tolbutamide.
- Postprandial glucose regulators, including nateglinide and repaglinide
- Alpha-glucosidase inhibitors – the only alpha-glucosidase inhibitor currently licensed in the UK is acarbose (brand name Glucobay)
- Biguanides – metformin is now the only one available.
- Thiazolidinediones (glitazones), including pioglitazone and rosiglitazone

Sulphonylureas

The sulphonylureas were the very first non-insulin drugs used to treat diabetes. They were discovered by accident after scientists working on a treatment for typhoid noticed that a compound in the drug lowered blood glucose levels. As a result, the first sulphonylurea specifically developed to treat diabetes was introduced in 1956, although modern sulphonylureas are much more effective than the earlier forms.

Sulphonylureas reduce blood glucose by stimulating the beta cells in the pancreas to produce more insulin, whether or not you've had anything to eat. They'll cause your pancreas to keep releasing insulin all day, so if you miss a meal or if your meal doesn't contain enough carbohydrate, the extra insulin could make your blood glucose go too low, causing hypoglycaemia (see page 66). So if you're taking sulphonylureas, it's very important to eat regular, carbohydrate-based meals and snacks. It's not uncommon to suffer the odd hypo when you first start taking sulphonylureas, but your doctor will monitor this and with careful control of your diet and a reduction in dosage if necessary, sulphonylureas should keep your diabetes under control. Most sulphonylureas should be taken once a day with breakfast, although this depends on the individual medicine you've been prescribed.

Side effects

Sulphonylureas are not suitable for everybody, and may not be prescribed for those who are already overweight as one of the possible side effects is weight gain, due to the effects of the extra insulin. They can also, as already mentioned, cause hypos, but this may settle down after adjustments to the dose.

Postprandial glucose regulators (PPGRs)

PPGRs work in the same way as sulphonylureas by stimulating the pancreas to produce more insulin. The main difference is that PPGRs work more quickly and for a shorter period of time than sulphony-lureas – you take them before a meal, they stimulate the pancreas to produce insulin to cope with the glucose produced by that meal, then they stop working. As a result, they are less likely to cause a hypo. You only need to take PPGRs when you eat, so if you miss a meal, you don't need to take the drug. This means that there's no need to eat when you're not hungry. Both nateglinide and repaglinide should usually be taken around 30 minutes before meals.

Side effects

Side effects are rare with nateglinide and repaglinide, but some people may experience hypos, digestive upsets or flu-like symptoms.

Alpha-glucosidase inhibitors

Acarbose (Glucobay), the only alpha-glucosidase inhibitor licensed in the UK, works by slowing down the absorption of starch from the intestine. The carbohydrates we eat need to be broken down into simple sugar molecules so that the body can absorb them. The enzyme responsible for this process is alpha-glucosidase, which is found in the lining of the small intestine. Acarbose blocks the action of this enzyme, delaying the absorption of sugar molecules and thereby avoiding the sharp rise in blood glucose that may be experienced after a meal. Acarbose tablets should be swallowed just before a meal or chewed with the first mouthful of food.

Side effects

Arcobose has few side effects and is less likely to cause hypoglycae-mia than some of the other drugs. However, it does have one rather nasty side effect – flatulence. This occurs because the action of the drug means that there may be undigested starch lying around in the gut after a meal. This begins to ferment as is comes into contact with intestinal bacteria, and the result is flatulence and other digestive problems such as abdominal pain and diarrhoea. In most cases, these symptoms settle down and disappear after a month or two. Whether or not you continue with the drug will depend on whether you can tolerate the side effects at the start of treatment. You should not take acarbose if you have existing bowel problems such as inflammatory bowel disease or colonic ulceration.

Biguanides

Metformin is the only drug in this group now available. It works by reducing the amount of glucose produced by the cells in the liver, by improving the body's response to insulin, thereby increasing the body's uptake of glucose and reducing the absorption of glucose from the gut after eating, all of which result in lower blood glucose. Metformin is often the first choice of treatment for people who are overweight because it works as an appetite suppressant and may cause some weight loss. It can also reduce cholesterol levels. Metformin should be taken with food in order to minimize side effects.

Side effects

Side effects are fairly common with metformin and are experienced by around 30 per cent of those who take it. Again these tend to be digestive upsets such as nausea, vomiting, diarrhoea, abdominal pain and loss of appetite. Some people are able to control these effects by taking the drug with meals, and by starting with a small dose and gradually increasing it. A rare but very serious complication is lactic acidosis, which can be fatal. An early biguanide, pheformin, was taken off the market because of this side effect. Poor liver or kidney function can be a factor in lactic acidosis, so you should not take metformin if you have any signs of either, or if you have heart failure or drink a lot of alcohol.

Thiazolidinediones

The name for this group of drugs is a bit of a mouthful, so they're often referred to as the glitazones, which although it sounds rather like a 1970s Glam Rock band, is considerably easier to say than thiazolidinediones! The glitazones include pioglitazone and rosiglitazone, both of which were launched in 2000, so they're still fairly new. Another glitazone, troglitazone, (brand name Rezulin) was withdrawn from the market after more than 60 people using it suffered fatal liver damage. Glitazones work by reducing insulin resistance and improving the body's sensitivity to its own insulin, helping it to use the natural supply more effectively. Glitazones can be taken with or without food but should be taken at the same time each day.

Side effects

Side effects are minimal with glitazones. They include weight gain, swollen ankles, anaemia and tiredness. The newer glitazones are thought to be unlikely to cause liver problems and, at the time of writing, published clinical trials have indicated no adverse effects on the liver. However, it is recommended that liver function tests should be carried out before treatment begins, every two months for the first year of treatment and then periodically from then on. Liver function tests involve a blood sample being taken and sent to the laboratory for testing. On the plus side, there is evidence to suggest that glitazones may have a positive effect on blood pressure and other cardiovascular risk factors.

Combinations of drugs

If the drug you have been prescribed doesn't work at all or isn't effective enough, your doctor may suggest combining two or even three different drugs to keep your blood glucose under control. For example, you might be prescribed metformin to prevent your liver from producing too much glucose, but if this doesn't reduce your blood glucose levels sufficiently, a glitazone may be added to counter insulin resistance. You may find that a particular drug or combination of drugs works perfectly for years, but then becomes ineffective. If this happens, your doctor may suggest insulin, either in combination with tablets or on its own. The advantage of starting insulin as part of a combination therapy along with tablets is that it gives you a chance to get used to injecting insulin and also to adjust the dose according to your blood glucose readings (see page 70).

Insulin

Insulin may be necessary for the treatment of type 2 diabetes when a combination of diet, exercise and drug therapy fails to control your blood glucose adequately. If your blood glucose levels have been high for some time as a result of insulin resistance, there is a good chance that your beta cells (the insulin-producing cells in your pancreas) have become worn out from trying to compensate (see Chapter 1). As a result, you may suffer a return of symptoms such as thirst, tiredness and itchiness, especially in the genital area. The decision to move to insulin may be a bit scary, especially if you're concerned about being able to give yourself injections, but try not to worry – the vast majority of people with type 2 diabetes who change to insulin treatment report a considerable improvement in general well-being. The most important thing is that your blood glucose is kept under control – study after study has concluded that keeping blood glucose as near normal as possible is the single most important factor in avoiding the serious complications of diabetes. If your doctor decides you need to switch to insulin, your treatment may continue to be managed by your GP, or it may be supervised by the hospital from that point onwards, or it may be managed by both your GP and the hospital, depending on where you live.

Insulin was discovered back in 1921 in Canada. Researchers found that by injecting a primitive form of insulin into a dog whose pancreas had been removed, they were able to keep the animal alive even though it produced no insulin of its own. Early forms were made from the pancreases of cows and pigs. We still use some bovine and porcine insulin today, although 'human insulin', which is produced in the laboratory by genetic engineering, is more widely used.

Different types of insulin

There are several different types of insulin, all of which have different absorption rates and peaks of activity. The type most suitable for you will depend on how your body responds to insulin and how you want to use it. It may take a period of trial and error before you find the best type of insulin and dosing schedule to fit in with your lifestyle, but you should be able to discuss this with your diabetes health-care team.

- Rapid-acting analogue insulin – the main advantage is that this insulin can be used just before eating, with food or just after food. It's a fast-onset insulin which peaks very quickly and can last from two to five hours. It may not last quite long enough to control your blood glucose levels from one meal to the next, so it may need to be mixed with a longer-acting insulin.
- Long-acting analogue insulin – different from other insulins in that it is absorbed slowly so that the effects last longer. It should be used once a day, at the same time each day, and should last for around 24 hours. This may be suitable for those who are elderly or frail or for those who rely on someone else to give them their injections.
- Short-acting, also known as soluble insulin – this works quickly to counter the rise in blood glucose experienced after eating and should be used about 15–30 minutes before meals. Its peak action occurs within two to six hours and it can last for up to eight hours.
- Medium- and long-acting insulins – these work over several hours to keep your blood glucose under control between meals and are usually taken half an hour before meals or before bed. They can last from between eight and 30 hours, with their peak activity occurring at between four and 12 hours. They may be used in conjunction with short-acting insulins.
- Insulin mixtures – combinations of short- and longer-acting insulins in various proportions. These are used 15–30 minutes before eating to cope with the rise in blood glucose that occurs after eating. The longer-acting portion continues to work between meals.

Side effects

Some people can experience a slight itching or swelling around the injection site when they first start using insulin, but this usually disappears within a few weeks. Very occasionally, someone will have an allergic reaction to one of the added components in insulin, such as a preservative. This can be remedied by using another insulin that does not contain that particular additive. The only other side effect of insulin in hypoglycaemia, which can occur if too much insulin is injected, thus causing blood glucose levels to fall too low. This is more likely to be a problem when you first start on insulin, and although you should constantly be aware of the warning signs, it usually settles down once the correct dose has been established. Bear in mind that you may need to use more or less insulin than usual if you eat more or less than you'd planned or if you exercise more or less than you'd planned. The dose may also need to be adjusted if you become ill or stressed.

Symptoms of hypoglycaemia

You need to be able to recognize the signs of a hypo if you get them (not everybody does) so that you can take action immediately. An untreated hypo can seriously impair brain function, leading to extreme confusion, seizures, delirium and loss of consciousness. Symptoms vary from person to person, but common warning signs are:

- Feeling faint or dizzy
- Loss of co-ordination
- Headache
- Blurred vision
- Feeling hungry
- Feeling weak and shaky
- Sweating
- Palpitations
- Feeling anxious or irritable
- Mental confusion

If you notice any of these signs, have something sweet immediately, for example, half a glass of fruit juice or a fizzy drink, a handful or raisins or two teaspoons of honey. Depending on when your next meal is due, you may need to follow this up with a starchy snack to keep you going.

If you are unable to treat the hypo yourself – if, for example, you didn't recognize the warning signs and become too confused to know what to do – it may be possible for a family member or friend to give you a glucogen injection. Glucogen is a natural hormone that raises blood glucose by stimulating the liver to release glucose into the bloodstream. It may be worth keeping a glucogen injection kit on hand if you know you are prone to hypos but don't recognize them (or don't experience any symptoms in advance). You should also wear or carry some form of identification that says you have diabetes that is controlled by insulin or tablets. That way, if you become confused or are unable to communicate, anyone who finds you will be able to see that you're suffering from a complication of diabetes and seek appropriate help (see Chapter 9).

One of the problems with using insulin is that, with blood glucose control being generally very good, the body may get used to quite low blood glucose levels, which can mean you don't get the usual hypo warning signs. If this happens, your doctor may suggest that you raise your levels very slightly for up to three months, simply to re-sensitize your body to hypo symptoms.

Giving yourself an injection

You won't relish the idea of having to stick a needle into yourself once a day or maybe more often, but you'll be shown how to do it and in no time you'll become an expert at injecting your dose of insulin quickly and painlessly. Needles and syringes are much easier to use than they used to be, and modern needles are now so fine that you can hardly feel the injection.

How to inject yourself

Your diabetes nurse or another member of your health-care team will show you how it's done and will watch you practise until you have it right, but here are a few tips to make the process easier and more efficient.

- Don't clean the injection site with alcohol or spirit as this can make the injection sting. Soap and water is fine, although you may not really need to clean the skin every time you inject (unless you work on a building site or if you've not been taking baths or showers!).
- Pinch the skin with your fingers and insert the needle diagonally so it slides in just beneath the skin but not into the muscle.
- When you have injected the insulin, release the skin and pull the needle out.
- If bleeding occurs, press the site gently until it stops, but don't rub the area.

However, injections can be difficult for some people – for example those with a needle phobia or those with arthritis, who may find manouvering the needle rather a problem. Unfortunately, we still don't have an insulin pill. Scientists are still trying to find a way to give insulin by mouth, but at the moment this is not possible because it is destroyed by digestive acid in the gut. Other methods of administering insulin are the insulin pen, the insulin jet injector, and, soon to hit the market, the insulin inhaler.

Insulin pens

There are several different types of insulin pen, but they all work in the same way. They look like an ordinary, chunky pen. You set the amount of insulin you need, hold the pen against your skin and then you push a plunger or press a button to inject the insulin. Some types of pen are disposable, so you just throw them away when the insulin runs out, whereas others have a cartridge and you just replace each cartridge as it runs out.

Insulin jet injectors

These could be the answer if you have a needle phobia, and they are available on prescription. They work by using high-pressure air to send a fine jet of insulin through your skin. However, they may cause some bruising to the skin. Also, you have to boil these devices frequently to sterilize them.

Insulin inhalers

After more than seven years of successful trials, the insulin inhaler is, it is hoped, about to be licensed for general use. The inhaler contains a new powdered form of fast-acting insulin and can be puffed at mealtimes when insulin is most needed. It enters the bloodstream via the lungs and begins to work very quickly. However, people would still have to take a long-acting insulin injection. Scientists suggest that, for those with type 2 diabetes who are already on diabetes pills, the inhaler offers better blood glucose control than adding another type of tablet. The inhaler will make life much easier for those who find it difficult or inconvenient to inject insulin several times a day.

Insulin patches

Scientists have been trying to develop insulin patches for some time, although there has been little success. There are some products currently in development but it is not thought that these will be a real alternative in the near future.

Complementary medicines and therapies

Herbal supplements, food supplements and complementary therapies such as reflexology, aromatherapy and acupuncture have become increasingly popular over the past two decades. Many claim to help the symptoms of type 2 diabetes and its complications or, in some cases, to prevent or delay the onset of the disease. But one of the problems with complementary medicines is that most of them are not tested and regulated in the same way that other drugs are, so their efficacy is not certain; nor is it always possible to say whether they will interact with other medicines.

Many people are under the impression that herbal or nutritional supplements are natural, and therefore cannot be harmful. This is not so. Bear in mind that the earliest medicines were made from herbs or other naturally occurring substances and many still are. So just as you would check with your doctor or pharmacist whether it would be safe to take a certain medicine as well as those you are already taking, you should also check before taking any herbal or nutritional remedy. Also, bear in mind that some remedies and therapies could interact with the complications of diabetes.

There has been some interesting and encouraging research into the use of cinnamon, for example, which may improve blood glucose and blood fats in people with type 2 diabetes. However, large quantities of the spice can be toxic, so we need more research on the subject.

The karela plant, traditionally used in Asian cookery, is also known to reduce blood glucose levels. However, karela capsules are being widely advertised as a treatment for diabetes, and Diabetes UK is concerned that this advertising is misleading. The charity warns that karela capsules are an unknown entity and it has issued a statement to this effect on its website:

> ... while certain components of karela do have hypoglycaemic effects there have been no formal studies to indicate if it can be used safely in capsule form by people with diabetes. Many natural products and herbal medicines are not safe when used in conjunction with other pharmaceutical medicines and can cause problems. As there is a lack of information both on the concentration of karela in these capsules and the effects of other

components Diabetes UK does not recommend their use until further evidence is available about their use in the management of diabetes.

While it is sensible to treat complementary medicines with as much caution as you would any other drug, this doesn't mean that all vitamins, supplements, remedies, therapies or treatments are bad and should be avoided at all costs. It may be the case that some supplements help to control blood glucose levels, and there is some anecdotal evidence to suggest that reflexology can stimulate the pancreas to work more efficiently. There is no doubt that there are some therapies that can help you feel more relaxed and can generally improve your quality of life. But it cannot be stressed highly enough that no supplement, remedy or therapy should take the place of diet, exercise and prescribed medication. You should always check with both your doctor and the appropriate (qualified) herbalist, therapist or practitioner before embarking on a course of complementary treatment.

All about testing

Testing your blood glucose levels is an excellent way of taking control of your condition and managing your blood glucose. There is a great deal of evidence to suggest that keeping tight control of your blood glucose levels is the most effective way to reduce the risks of the serious complications of diabetes. You should try to keep levels as near normal as possible, that is, 4–7 mmol/l before meals and no more than 10 mmol/l after meals. Testing allows you to monitor the effectiveness of your diet and exercise regime and of any medication you're using, and it also enables you to make lifestyle changes as necessary to try and lower your levels if they start to creep up.

Whether and how often you test is up to you and your diabetes health-care team, so it's important to understand the benefits and drawbacks as well as the process and types of testing. It's important to make sure you carry out the test properly or you may get inaccurate results. You also need to be able to understand exactly what the results mean.

If you control your diabetes by diet and exercise alone, you may feel that having a regular HbA1c (glycated haemoglobin) test is enough. This is a test that should be carried out by your doctor at least once a year, but preferably every three to six months. The test is a simple blood test that looks at your general blood glucose control to give an idea of how your diabetes management is working overall. Ideally, your HbA1c should be below 7 per cent.

If you use insulin, it's more important to test yourself regularly because testing can alert you to low blood glucose levels as well as high, and insulin can cause your levels to fall dangerously low.

Urine testing

Although the purpose of testing is to check the level of glucose in your blood, high levels will also show up in your urine. In fact, ancient Greek doctors diagnosed the disease by tasting the urine of their patients, while the more squeamish Chinese would get the patient to urinate on a flat stone and then watch to see whether the urine drew a stampede of sugar-hungry ants.

Basically, when your blood glucose levels become too high, glucose spills out into your urine as the body frantically tries to rid itself of the excess sugar. Some doctors argue that urine testing isn't accurate enough, and because of this, you may find it difficult to get testing strips on prescription in some areas. Urine testing may be suitable if you manage your diabetes with diet and exercise alone, or if the only medication you take is metformin. It is not suitable for those on insulin or any medication that may cause hypoglycaemia because urine testing cannot tell you that your blood glucose is too low. The other disadvantage is that the test can only tell you that your blood glucose was high when the urine was being produced, which may be several hours earlier. If you opt for urine testing, it's very important to make sure you get regular HbA1c tests so that you can keep an eye on the overall picture.

To carry out a urine test, dip a test strip into a sample of urine and then check for colour changes to the strip by holding it against the side of the strip container and matching the colour against the range shown. Any colour change usually indicates that there is glucose in your urine. How often you test should be discussed with your diabetes care team, but many people who use urine testing find that testing on two days a week is sufficient. On those days, they carry out a test before each meal. A positive test means that your blood glucose is probably more than 10 mmol/l and you should be aiming for 7 mmol/l before meals.

If you find that your levels are going over 7 mmol/l or that your HbA1c goes over 7 per cent, this is an indication that your control is not as good as it could be. If this happens only occasionally and for a reason you're aware of – maybe you've been to a wedding or some other celebration and you've eaten more than usual – a re-adjustment of your diet should sort things out. However, it's a good idea to keep a record of your test results and anything that could affect them, such as illness or a special occasion, so that you can see whether you need to take further action. If you can't think of any reason why you've had a positive test, or you have several positive tests, you should discuss this with your doctor. It may be that you need to start on tablets for your diabetes, or if you're on metformin, you may need to increase the dose.

Testing your blood

This is a much more accurate way to test your blood glucose levels and will also show when levels are falling too low as well as rising too high. To carry out the test you'll need to wash and dry your hands thoroughly, then obtain a drop of blood by pricking your finger with a disposable lancet – a short, very fine needle. This may be uncomfortable until you get the hang of it, but with practice, you'll barely feel it. Most people prefer to prick the side of the finger rather than the fingerprint area, which has more sensitive nerve endings. If you don't get a good droplet of blood, rubbing the finger up and down a few times should help. Place the blood onto a test strip, then read and record the results, which may be read visually or with a blood glucose meter.

Choosing and using a meter

There are many different meters on the market and your health-care team will help you to decide which one is best for you. You might want to consider the size and weight of the meter, especially if you need to carry it in a pocket or handbag. Will you write down your readings each time, or would a meter that remembers your readings be more useful? Although you should read through the set of instructions very carefully yourself, your health-care team should also be able help you to learn how to use your meter. You need to know whether your meter measures whole blood (the blood as it comes out of your finger) or plasma (the substance remaining after red and white blood cells and platelets have been removed). If your meter measures whole blood glucose, the results may be slightly lower than those you would get on a meter that was set up to measure plasma.

To make sure your readings are accurate, it's important to check regularly that the meter is still working properly. Most meters come with a small bottle of control solution that you can use to check whether your meter is giving reliable results. You may also get an inaccurate reading if the blood sample is too small, if the sample is contaminated, if your testing strips are out of date or have been stored incorrectly, or if you are using the meter incorrectly. Modern meters are fairly simple to use, but mistakes – such as unwittingly calling up a previous reading – do happen!

How often should you test?

If you've recently been diagnosed and use insulin or are taking sulphonylurea tablets, you may need to test around four times a day, before meals and before bed. Once you manage to take close control of your levels and they become more stable, you'll probably be able to reduce the number of tests.

Many people test between two and four times a day on two or three days a week. If you test at different times of the day, you'll get a clearer picture of how your levels are changing. If you're not on insulin or sulphonylureas, you could try testing twice a day, two or three times a week, going down to twice a week at different times once things are more stable.

You should test frequently if you are unwell, because illness can cause considerable fluctuation in your blood glucose levels. If your levels are up, report this to your doctor – you may need to increase the dose of any diabetes medication you are using. You should also test before and after exercise, when you start a new medication that might affect your blood glucose, and, if you're taking insulin or some other diabetes medications, before driving and if you're pregnant. (See Chapter 8 for more about pregnancy and diabetes.)

As with urine testing, you should keep a written record of your test results so that you can spot any fluctuations in your levels or trends towards higher levels. This enables you and your health-care team to make changes to your care plan. Even if you manage your diabetes with diet and exercise alone, you can make small changes that may improve your levels. For example, if one day you have a reading of 12 mmol/l, you could go for a walk or do some gardening or whatever to bring those levels down. You should also think about why the levels may have risen. Has there been a special occasion where you ate a bigger meal than usual? Have you forgotten to take your medication? Have you been ill? These are all reasons that your levels may have gone up. If you can identify a reason, it can help put you on guard against anything similar happening in future. If there's no apparent reason, it may be that you need a change in treatment.

Not all people who have type 2 diabetes regularly test their own blood glucose levels. It should be a choice that you make once you have all the relevant information. There's no doubt that testing can be a very useful diabetes management tool, but some people really don't want to test because they feel it's a constant reminder of their diabetes. Others don't write down the results for fear of being 'told off' by their health-care team if the results are too high, or they even make up the results to make them look 'better' or to avoid doing the test. This means that they can't be given appropriate advice on controlling their condition – and as the results are meaningless, it's a waste of time, too! If you're unhappy or unsure about home testing, talk it over with your health-care team – they may be able to put your mind at rest, or they may agree that testing isn't right for you.

Why it's worth the hassle

Testing your blood or urine (or both), injecting insulin, taking pills and watching what you eat can all seem too much from time to time, especially as it emphasizes the fact that you have diabetes. Some people can be tempted to let things slip or just ignore the whole thing in the hope that it might go away. It won't!

Keith, aged 50, was diagnosed eight years ago. He now takes 16 tablets a day, three different liquid medicines, vitamin and herb supplements (prescribed by an NHS-recommended herbalist) and has eight or nine insulin injections each day.

'I actually asked to go on insulin three years ago,' says Keith. 'But the doctor I was seeing at the time dismissed the idea, saying that most of his patients would do anything to stay off it, so why was I so keen to start using it? I just wanted to get well. I'd had diabetes for some time before I was diagnosed. I'd had a few health problems, but like most blokes, I don't like going to the doctor and, having been told as a youngster that the pain I had from a perforated bowel was 'psychosomatic', I've learned to keep quiet about any problems. I eventually went to the doctor about fatty lumps that had appeared on my elbow (probably due to high triglyceride levels). They tested my blood and urine and phoned me two hours later to say I was diabetic. They put me on lots of medication but my blood sugar levels just wouldn't come down, and I ended up in hospital for about four weeks. I was given lots of advice on diet, and I realized I'd become addicted to sugar – I'd eat one meal a day and fill up with Mars bars, biscuits and so on. They also said I needed to test my blood glucose regularly and record the results. I did this meticulously, and the readings were still high even though I was very careful with my diet. I'd lost a few kilograms in weight but I wasn't feeling any better. When I took my records back to the hospital and showed the doctor, he wrote 'faulty monitor' on my notes. Basically, the levels were so high, he didn't believe they were accurate. Last year I saw a different doctor who was appalled that this had been ignored. He agreed I should start on insulin immediately and I've never looked back. I have to inject several times a day, and yes, it does worry me that one day the insulin will stop working. But in the meantime, I'm finally starting to feel better.

It's a pain having to inject and do so much testing, but I'd rather have the inconvenience of that than end up having a heart attack or losing a leg. I know I'm very ill. I don't like it, and I don't like to think that, at 50, I've already had to retire. But the most important thing is to stay healthy, so I don't care how many pills, tests, injections and so on I have to deal with, as long as I can stay as healthy as possible and get the most out of my life.'

8

Pregnancy and diabetes

It used to be extremely unusual for type 2 diabetes to develop in those aged under 40, and so concerns about pregnancy were unlikely to be necessary. However, a report by Diabetes UK stated that were almost 100,000 people aged 15–44 years in the UK with type 2 diabetes in 2004. As time goes on, more and more younger people are being diagnosed, so it's as well to know of the possible problems someone with type 2 might experience in pregnancy. If you're male, your diabetes won't affect your partner's pregnancy (nor will it affect her chances of conceiving – diabetes does not affect your sperm count). If you're female and are planning to become pregnant, it's very important to make sure your blood glucose levels are under control before you become pregnant, because raised blood glucose early in pregnancy can cause birth defects.

The vast majority of mothers with diabetes (this includes type 1, type 2 and gestational diabetes) have normal, healthy pregnancies and deliver normal, healthy babies. However, if you have diabetes you are at increased risk of some of the common complications of pregnancy, such as high blood pressure, pre-eclampsia and prolonged or early labour, so this is another reason to take extra care before and during your pregnancy.

Preparing for a healthy pregnancy

The first eight weeks after conception are crucial in the baby's development, so make sure you keep tight control of your blood glucose levels before becoming pregnant as well as throughout your pregnancy. Frequent testing (see Chapter 7) will help you to monitor your levels.

As soon as you know you are pregnant or, preferably, as soon as you decide to become pregnant, you should ask your diabetes care team for advice on how your treatment should proceed during your pregnancy, what tests you may need and so on. You may need to change your diet and medication. If possible, arrange to see an endocrinologist or an obstetrician who is experienced in treating women with diabetes. It would also be good to see a diabetes dietician who specializes in pregnancy, but in the meantime, try to follow these basic guidelines:

- Stop smoking – smoking increases your risk of miscarriage, premature delivery and stillbirth, and it can also cause birth defects and developmental problems in your unborn child. Smoking causes even more problems for people with diabetes, significantly increasing your risk of complications such as high blood pressure. If you're having trouble stopping, ask your doctor or midwife for help.
- Avoid alcohol – the advice to pregnant women used to be to drink alcohol in moderation, however, there is increasing evidence to suggest that the safest option is to avoid alcohol completely during pregnancy.
- Be obsessive about your diet – get advice from a dietician and stick to it rigidly. This is the best way to keep control of your blood glucose levels.
- Have your eyes checked – especially if you are already experiencing eye problems or have been diagnosed with retinopathy. Pregnancy can increase the pressure on the small blood vessels in your eyes making them more prone to damage, so it's important to have your condition monitored by an opthalmologist.

It is recommended that women who are planning a pregnancy should start taking a folic acid supplement before trying to conceive and then for the first twelve weeks of pregnancy. Folic acid is a vitamin that helps prevent the baby from developing neural tube defects, including spina bifida. Some doctors advise women with diabetes to take a slightly higher dose than those who don't have diabetes. You should discuss this with your diabetes care team.

If you are taking any medication for your diabetes or for any related or non-related condition, discuss this with your doctor before you become pregnant, since some medicines, especially tablets for diabetes or for high blood pressure, can damage the developing fetus.

Treatment during pregnancy

If you're already on tablets for your diabetes, you may need to switch to insulin until after the birth. (See page 64 for more about insulin treatment.) You can usually go back to tablets after your baby is born. Even if you usually control your diabetes with diet and exercise alone, you may find that you need to use insulin in the later stages of pregnancy, because insulin resistance tends to increase around that time. After your baby has been born, insulin resistance will quickly return to your pre-pregnancy level.

Gestational diabetes mellitus

Gestational diabetes mellitus (GDM) is the name given to a form of diabetes that occurs during, and as a result of, pregnancy. It isn't strictly speaking type 2 diabetes, but developing it while pregnant does mean you're more likely to develop type 2 diabetes in later life – between 40 and 50 per cent of women who have GDM will develop type 2 diabetes within 15–20 years after giving birth. Pregnancy effects blood glucose levels even in women who do not have diabetes, so there is some debate among doctors as to how high the levels should be for a diagnosis of gestational diabetes to be made.

During pregnancy, extra hormones are produced that prevent naturally produced insulin from working efficiently in the body. In most women, the pancreas simply steps up insulin production and everything is fine. But if the pancreas cannot produce enough extra insulin to counter this effect, blood glucose levels rise and diabetes is diagnosed. GDM is a temporary form of the disease. It usually develops during the second half of pregnancy and disappears completely soon after the birth. However, it may be that you should consider it an early warning sign, because it suggests that you don't have much 'pancreatic reserve'. Although your pancreas copes with your insulin needs on a day-to-day basis, it cannot produce enough to cope with the extra demand put on it by pregnancy. This means that if your pancreatic reserve is not great enough to cope with extra stresses that occur in the future – illness, for example, or increased insulin resistance due to overweight – you are likely to develop type 2 diabetes. For the same reason, having GDM in one pregnancy increases the risk of developing it in subsequent pregnancies. You can reduce the risk, both of GDM and of type 2 diabetes, by losing weight if you need to and following a sensible diet and exercise programme (see Chapters 5 and 6).

Very occasionally, tests in pregnancy reveal that the woman is already suffering from type 1 or type 2 diabetes. This is different from GDM and will need to continue to be treated after the birth.

Risk factors for GDM:

Risk factors for gestational diabetes include:

- Having a family history of type 2 diabetes
- Having GDM in a previous pregnancy
- Being over 25–30 years of age
- Having previously given birth to a large baby (over 9 pounds or 4 kilograms)
- Having previously suffered an unexplained stillbirth
- Being significantly overweight

Diagnosing GDM

Few women notice any symptoms of GDM. You may be hungrier or thirstier than usual, and you may need to pass urine more frequently, but since these symptoms are common in later pregnancy anyway, you may not notice anything amiss.

GDM is usually picked up by a blood or urine test between 24 and 28 weeks of pregnancy. Urine is routinely tested throughout pregnancy and if glucose is found, you'll probably be given a glucose tolerance test (GTT) to check the levels of glucose in your blood. You may also be offered this test if you are considered to have a high risk of developing GDM. The GTT involves fasting for six hours before attending a special clinic where the test will be carried out. Your blood will be tested when you first arrive. This will measure your blood glucose level after you've been fasting and is called a baseline test. You'll then be asked to drink a sweet, sugary mixture after which your blood will be tested at set intervals and the measurements compared with the normal range. Remember that most women who have glucose in their urine at their antenatal appointment turn out to have normal blood glucose levels in the glucose tolerance test.

Treating GDM

The treatment for GDM is much the same as for type 2, except that diabetes tablets can't be taken. The aim of treatment is to keep blood glucose levels as near to normal as possible, and for many women, diet and exercise is enough to achieve this. Your doctor or dietician will advise you on what sort of foods to choose and how much you should be eating (see Chapter 5), and you may be advised to test your blood glucose, either by testing your urine or by using a blood glucose monitor (see Chapter 7). Ask your doctor or midwife for advice on suitable exercise during pregnancy. You should aim to exercise gently but regularly – walking is perfect and will help you feel more healthy and energetic as well as helping to reduce your blood glucose levels.

If diet and exercise isn't enough to keep your levels under control, you will need to have insulin injections. Don't worry too much about this – around 10–30 per cent of women with GDM use insulin until blood glucose returns to normal, usually very soon after the birth. Your levels will probably be tested after delivery and at your six-week post-natal check to make sure.

Effects of GDM on the baby and the birth

Because GDM tends to develop in the second trimester, by which time the baby's major organs are fairly well developed, the risk to the baby is lower than in those with type 1 or type 2 diabetes. However, if it transpires that diabetes was already present before the pregnancy, there may be an increased risk of birth defects, the extent of which depends on how high the blood glucose levels were and for how long.

Raised blood glucose can result in a very big baby, which does slightly increase the risk of injury to both mother and baby during the birth. Your baby's development and growth will be carefully monitored if you have GDM, and if the baby appears to be very large, your doctors may suggest inducing labour at around 38–39 weeks, possibly by planned Caesarean section to avoid complications and the need for an emergency Caesarean delivery.

After your baby has been born, doctors will keep an eye on his or her blood glucose levels to make sure they're not too low. This is because the baby's pancreas made extra insulin in response to your high blood glucose levels and may continue to do so even for a short while after the birth. If this happens, a glucose solution may be given intravenously to stabilize the levels.

Research suggests that the children of mothers who have diabetes, including GDM, are more likely to develop diabetes themselves.

In almost all cases, GDM disappears after the birth. But if you do develop it, take action straight away to keep your levels under control, to reduce the risk of it developing in subsequent pregnancies and to reduce your risk of developing type 2 diabetes.

9

Living with type 2 diabetes

So far, we've looked mainly at the physical aspects of type 2 diabetes, particularly in terms of trying to prevent or delay its onset, and in terms of managing the condition once it is diagnosed. But if you or someone close has recently been diagnosed, you'll be aware that the physical side is only part of what you have to come to terms with. There are also psychological, social and practical considerations to take into account, and this chapter looks at some of those aspects of living with diabetes.

Coping with depression

People with diabetes, especially women, are more likely to suffer from depression than people who don't have the disease, but what is not yet certain is why this is so. Some studies suggest that there is a physical link between depression and diabetes, but there is no firm evidence to support this. It has also been suggested that those who develop depression already have a tendency to the illness even before they're diagnosed with diabetes. But what is known for certain is that depression can occur as a result of trauma and distress, and a diagnosis of an incurable illness can indeed be traumatic and distressing. In fact, people diagnosed with diabetes may pass through similar stages to those who have been bereaved: disbelief, denial, anger and depression.

Whether your depression is due to physical or psychological factors, it's important to recognize that depression is a serious, potentially life-threatening illness in itself, whether you have diabetes or not. If you have diabetes as well, depression can affect the way you manage your diabetes. For example, if you have depression, you're less likely to take physical exercise and more likely to under- or overeat with little regard to the effects on your blood glucose, you may forget or not bother to take your medication, and you're more likely to smoke or drink too much alcohol. These behaviours can in turn lead to increased risk of diabetes complications.

The term 'depression' is one that is overused and often misused. As a result many people misunderstand the illness and fail to take it seriously. This may explain the stigma that seems to exist in the UK, and would explain why sufferers are often reluctant to seek treatment.

What is depression?

There is a huge difference between being depressed and simply feeling 'a bit down'. It's often easier to recognize the signs in someone else than in yourself, so if you think you may be at risk – if you've had depression in the past, for example – talk to your family and friends about it. That way, they can be alert to any signs and symptoms that you might miss.

We all feel low sometimes, and knowing that you have diabetes can make you feel very low. After all, your life will change forever. You may have to drastically change your lifestyle, you may be worrying about entering the world of doctors' surgeries and hospital clinics for the first time, or you may have just learned that you will have to take medication for the rest of your life. Each of these is unsettling. You may feel quite miserable about it all and you have every right to. In normal circumstances, you would gradually start to feel less sad as you discovered more about your illness and treatment, and eventually you would go back to having the odd 'off' day like most people. However, if you continue to feel very sad, bleak or hopeless for longer than a few days, you may have depression.

The manifestation of the illness varies from person to person, but these are some of the signs to look out for:

- Persistent low mood, often worse in the mornings, improving as the day goes on
- Tearfulness
- Feeling unable to experience pleasure or enjoyment
- Loss of interest in social and work activities
- Reduced or increased appetite
- Sleep difficulties – sleeplessness or early morning wakening, or markedly increased need for sleep
- Lack of energy, fatigue
- Slowed thinking, speech or movements

- Inability to concentrate
- Anxiety, panic attacks
- Feelings of worthlessness and hopelessness
- Being able to only see the negative side of things
- Suicidal thoughts and ideas

You don't need to experience all of these symptoms to have depression, and indeed some of them may be more to do with your diabetes, but if you think it may be depression, talk to your doctor about treatment. It is no good telling someone with depression to 'cheer up' or 'pull yourself together'. If you have depression, the chemicals in your brain that govern your mood make it impossible for you to simply elevate your mood – it's like telling someone with a broken leg to run for a bus. Like diabetes, depression is a serious illness that requires treatment, possibly with medication, counselling, cognitive behaviour therapy or a combination of these. Self-help books may also be useful, in fact a 'books-on-prescription' scheme launched in Devon in 2004 has had encouraging results (see page 112). The most important thing to remember is that, while depression or anxiety may be a normal reaction to a diagnosis of diabetes, this does not mean it will go away by itself. It might, but it probably won't. The good news is that it can be successfully treated in the majority of cases. It may take several months or even a year or more, and if you're treated with antidepressants, it's vital that you take them for at least six months after you last had symptoms. But not only will you feel better and be able to enjoy life once more, you'll also be better able to manage your diabetes, thus reducing the risk of complications.

Sexual difficulties

It is not uncommon for both men and women to experience sexual difficulties as a consequence of their diabetes. Sometimes these problems are physical complications of the disease, but we'll look at them in this chapter because sexual matters are so closely linked with emotional and psychological well-being. Whether your own sexual problems have a physical or psychological cause, you need to address them as soon as possible so that you can take steps to improve matters and to avoid any unnecessary problems developing in your relationship.

Erectile dysfunction

This is the most common problem experienced by men with diabetes. In fact, it is estimated that between 30 and 60 per cent of men with diabetes have problems achieving or maintaining an erection, or find that their erection is not strong enough to allow penetrative sex. This is often the result of damage to nerves and blood vessels that supply the penis. As we have seen, poor blood glucose control increases the risk of neuropathy and damage to blood vessels, so it is very important to keep a check on your glucose levels and to adjust your diet and exercise pattern if necessary. If you smoke, you're even more likely to become impotent because nicotine causes the blood vessels to constrict, reducing blood flow to the penis. Some types of medication, especially some blood pressure drugs and anti-depressants, may also cause erection problems and may affect your ability to have an orgasm. If these are possible side effects of any drug you're taking, talk to your doctor – it may be possible for you to switch to another drug.

There may also a psychological reason that you're having problems getting an erection. This could be linked to your feelings about your illness. Knowing that you have a serious, incurable illness can be very stressful, and negative stress can affect your ability to achieve an erection and your libido in general.

Loss of libido

Both men and women can experience a loss of libido as a result of diabetes. The root cause may be anxiety, fear, anger or depression. If you are overweight, low self-esteem or poor body image can also be a factor, so maybe tackling your weight could be a good starting point in helping you to feel like a sexual person again.

You may, as discussed earlier in this chapter, be suffering from depression, and this too can cause loss of libido as well as impotence. Sexual problems can also be one of the causes of depression, so it may be a question of working out which came first in order to find the most appropriate approach to treatment.

Female sexual problems

As well as loss of libido, women with diabetes may experience other sexual problems. High blood glucose levels increase the risk of neuropathy, which can cause reduced lubrication and painful intercourse as well as loss of sensation in the genital area, leading to difficulty in reaching orgasm. Yeast or urinary infections, which are also related to high blood glucose levels, can make intercourse painful and can affect the way you feel about your body and your ability to relax and enjoy intimate contact.

What can be done?

As with many of the complications of diabetes, sexual problems that have a physical cause, such as neuropathy, can be prevented or significantly reduced in severity by good control of bodyweight and blood glucose levels. However, you may need a little more help.

The most important thing to bear in mind is that, whatever the root cause of any sexual difficulty, it is a problem for the couple, not just for one partner. True, there may be physical aspects that need to be dealt with, and these may involve one partner taking a particular drug or using some medical device. But your sexual relationship with your partner is something you have created and nurtured between you, and any problems with it should have the attention of both partners.

Talk with your partner about what's happening in your sexual relationship and what bearing you feel that your diabetes may have. Are there physical difficulties such as erection problems? Vaginal dryness? Pain? Lack of sensation? Or do you think the problems may be more to do with how you feel about your illness and how it affects your sexuality? In many cases, one thing leads to the other. If sex is physically uncomfortable, you may find yourself avoiding sexual contact. This can make your partner think you're not interested, causing him or her to stop initiating sex, which in turn leads to you thinking your partner no longer finds you attractive. By this time, even if there is no underlying physical reason for the difficulties, and even if there is a spark of desire, you'll both be worrying so much that you're likely to experience some problems with arousal. Similarly, if you're worrying about how your illness affects you as a sexual person, and you lose confidence in your sexual ability, you may well find you have difficulty getting an erection. If you're a woman and you can't relax enough to become sufficiently aroused, you may find penetration painful, and so on.

By openly discussing sexual matters, you will be creating more intimacy, which can help heal the loss of confidence that is so closely linked with loss of libido. Many people find that this openess can stimulate their interest and desire. If you decide you need outside help, you will have already done some of the groundwork by discussing the problems with your partner, so hopefully you'll both be relaxed and comfortable with each other, and ready to tackle the problem together.

There are a number of options. The best place to start is probably your GP. Most doctors only allow a few minutes for each patient so book a double appointment so that you don't feel rushed. Your doctor may be able to offer advice, suggest a change in any medication you're already taking or prescribe a medicine or device that will help. Alternatively, he or she may refer you to a clinic specializing in psychosexual medicine. These clinics, which may be linked to the Family Planning Association, are staffed by doctors with a special interest and training in sexual difficulties.

Another option, especially if there is no underlying physical reason, is Relate. Although most people associate this organization with relationship counselling, Relate now offers help for sexual problems and has a number of trained psychosexual therapists. Relate usually makes a small charge for its services, based on what the client can afford. If you have access to the internet, Relate even offers online help with sexual problems. It may be tempting to take this route if you find it embarrassing to discuss your sex life with a stranger – and let's face it, who doesn't? – but try and remember that whoever is helping you with your problems is highly trained and has seen and heard it all before.

You may not be able to get help immediately. Relate usually has a waiting list and if your doctor refers you to a clinic, you may have to wait some time for an appointment. But don't put your sex life on hold until you've seen the right doctor or therapist or until you've taken the right pills. There is plenty you can do to keep things going while you're waiting. If there's no problem with desire, but your body refuses to do as it's told, forget about penetrative sex for a while and think in terms of other types of sexual contact.

If either or both of you have temporarily gone off sex, think instead about intimacy. If you can maintain some physical contact, it'll be easier to resume your sexual relationship once you are ready. Simply having a cuddle, holding hands or snuggling up together on the sofa can be reassuring and nourishing for your relationship. It may be a good idea to set boundaries – if one of you is not ready for sexual contact, you may want to be clear about no-go areas when you touch each other. Sometimes, just knowing that you're not going to have sex relieves the pressure enough to stimulate desire. In fact, one of the most successful ways of dealing with impotence (where there is no physical cause) is simply to ban sexual contact for a while – we always seem to want what we can't have!

Family and friends

The people closest to you can be a tremendous support and may be able to help practically as well, so it's probably best to keep them informed about your diabetes. You may find it difficult to talk about your illness, especially when you're first diagnosed – as we've already seen, many people go through a stage of denial before coming to terms with diabetes. Not wanting to talk about it is a similar reaction – a sort of 'if I ignore it, it might go away' mechanism.

Harvey was 46 when he was diagnosed 10 years ago. He didn't tell his wife for several days, and begged her not to tell their children or other family members. 'I felt guilty,' Harvey says. 'I was brought up to believe that the man was the breadwinner in a family. You have to stay strong no matter what. I was never one to go running up the doctor's at the slightest thing. In fact, I'd never been ill in my life – at that point, I hadn't had a single day off work in 26 years. I was a lorry driver then, although I had to retire early last year.

'They only found out I have diabetes by accident. My firm was bringing in a private health-care thing for employees and their families, and we had to have a medical when we signed up for it. They rang me at work the next day and told me there was sugar in my water and to go to my own doctor straight away. I couldn't bring myself to tell Joyce, my wife. I thought it must have been my fault I'd got this – all those doughnuts and chocolate bars I used to eat on the road. She guessed something was wrong in the end, so I had to tell her – she was imagining all sorts. Eventually she persuaded me to let her tell the kids, and they've been terrific about it, really supportive. My son helped me start exercising again – I was a few kilograms too heavy, to be honest, and sitting in that lorry all day didn't help. And my daughter's good as well – she's always phoning Joyce with different recipes and so on. They really look after me, my lot. I still find it hard not being totally fit, but Joyce has managed to convince me that it's not my fault and that I shouldn't feel guilty. She asked me how I would have felt if she'd been the one who was ill, had felt guilty and kept it quiet. She made her point!'

Some people find they have the opposite problem to Harvey. They want to talk about their diabetes, but find their friends and family unwilling to listen. This may be due to denial on their part. You won't want to force anyone to discuss your diabetes with you, but on the other hand, it can be dangerous to 'go along' with people who refuse to admit there's anything wrong. You have a serious illness, and it's an illness that can be managed well or allowed to run out of control, depending, in many cases, on the action taken (or not taken) by the person who has it. Of course your friends want you to be 'normal'; they would much rather you joined them in a slap-up meal with three courses including a big fat pudding, a few glasses of wine and a couple of brandies to go with the coffee and chocolate mints. They may be dismissive of your illness when you tell them you have to watch what you eat. 'Oh come on,' they say. 'One little lapse isn't going to hurt you.' Well, perhaps not, but it might. The truth is, one little lapse could lead to another or even another, and the combination of several 'little lapses', each of which may have sent your blood glucose soaring, could have a serious, long-lasting impact on your health.

On the other hand, you can find that people take on the role of 'food police', making themselves responsible for what you eat, and behaving as if they know best. Many people believe that those with diabetes should not eat any sugar at all, so they'll snatch a biscuit out of your hand and think they're doing you a favour! This sort of thing can be incredibly annoying, but they're probably acting out of genuine concern for your welfare. There are several ways of handling it. You can ignore it, in which case they'll probably get the message eventually, or you can explain in full, which can be tiresome if you have do it several times. Alternatively, you can try and do it with humour by adopting a tolerant smile and saying something like, 'and there I was thinking I should follow my doctor's advice!' Or you can thank them, say you are touched by their concern and that you really appreciate it, but you've worked very hard at learning about how to manage your condition by eating the right diet and you've now got it sorted.

You'll probably encounter a lot of ignorance when talking about your condition. That is not to say that other people are being deliberately obtuse and it is not meant to suggest that they are idiots. It is simply due to a lack of knowledge of, and therefore understanding of, diabetes. And frankly, why should they know anything about diabetes? Before you were diagnosed, you probably knew very little about it yourself. But it's now your job to educate those around you, especially those who may affect your diabetes or be affected by it, for example, people with whom you eat on a regular basis, especially those who may be preparing meals for you.

Diet is such an important part of diabetes management that you'll probably spend more time thinking about and talking about food than you ever have before. This can turn out to be one of the more positive things about having diabetes.

Alan, aged 58, a retired telecommunications manager, had never so much as boiled an egg before he was diagnosed. 'I'm embarrassed to admit it,' he says, 'but I've never been much of a "new man". My wife Norma always took care of shopping and cooking and so on, and the most I've ever done is make a bit of toast or heat up a can of beans. When I was diagnosed, I was referred to a dietician who spent a lot of time talking to me about healthy eating.

'I was always a bit of a pudding and pie man to be truthful, and I thought all salads were rabbit food. But the dietician went through the various food options with me, suggesting breakfasts and lunches that I'd never have thought of and even giving me a folder of recipes for healthy dinners.

'When I got home, I told Norma and we looked through the recipes together. She told me she'd never heard of some of the vegetables, and didn't know how to cook some of the meals, but she didn't seem bothered; she just said, "Oh well, we'll have to learn." And that's when I thought, well, if she can learn to cook something she's never cooked before, I suppose I can too. So I started taking more interest in food and Norma has taught me to cook – I don't think I ever would have learned had I not had diabetes!'

Alan's wife Norma is delighted with Alan's new interest in cooking. She says:

'To be perfectly honest, I was reluctant when he first talked about learning to cook. I didn't think he'd be any good at it and I thought I'd be able to do it quicker myself. But apart from making a right old mess in the kitchen, he's turned out to be a very good cook, and we both eat more healthily now. In fact, since he was diagnosed two years ago, I've lost over 10 kilograms! I still do the bulk of the cooking, but he regularly cooks the evening meal twice a week and he quite often does us a lovely salad for lunch during the week. We also help each other in the kitchen now – I'm his kitchen maid when he cooks and he's mine when I cook!'

So not only has Alan discovered a new hobby as a result of his diabetes, but it's also an activity that he and his wife now share and regard as fun, rather than a chore that was the responsibility of just one partner.

Employment

There is no reason why you should not find a job or continue with your current employment as long as your diabetes control is good, and you don't have complications that could affect your ability to work.

Will diabetes affect what jobs you can do?

Until recently, people with type 1 diabetes or with type 2 diabetes who use insulin were banned from working in the emergency services. Following some extensive campaigning by Diabetes UK, those blanket bans have now been lifted and anyone applying for a job with these services is subject to individual medical assessment. There are still some restrictions in place on people who want to be ambulance drivers or who want to drive large heavy goods vehicles or passenger-carrying vehicles. These restrictions are currently being challenged.

It used to be thought that people with diabetes should not do a job that involved shift work because this can affect your 'body clock', which means you might sleep and take your meals at unusual times, therefore making blood glucose control more difficult. These days, with better insulin programmes and improved glucose testing, you're more likely to be able to change the way you manage your diabetes without causing problems, so if you feel up to coping with shifts, talk to your diabetes care team about the best way to manage this.

Hazardous occupations

There are some occupations that, in certain circumstances, could present problems for someone with diabetes. If your vision is impaired because of retinopathy, for example, you might not be able to do a job that requires you to drive. If you regularly suffer hypos but don't get warning signs, it would be dangerous for you to be a firefighter. In many cases, though, it is possible to work quite safely in a potentially hazardous occupation. Diabetes UK has issued a list of guidelines to help employers and potential employees decide whether it would be safe for them to do hazardous jobs. Contact Diabetes UK (see page 109) for information about their booklet *Employment and Diabetes* and for a list of their other useful information booklets.

Applying for a job

Some employers ask you to complete a health questionnaire when applying for a job, or there is a section about health on the application form. If you are asked about any medical conditions, you must tell them about your diabetes. But if your condition is well controlled, you can say so on your application form, e.g. 'Type 2 diabetes, well controlled with diet/insulin/tablets.'

If you're not asked specifically, then you do not have to tell them. However, once you have been formally offered the appointment in writing, you may want to make them aware of your condition for a number of reasons. For example, you may need to arrange to take a few moments each day to inject your insulin, take your medication or test your blood glucose. There may be occasions when you need to have a snack very quickly. If you explain that you know how to manage your condition effectively, it should not affect their final decision. Indeed, if they then withdrew their offer and you suspected it was because of your diabetes, you may have a case under the Disability Discrimination Act (see below).

If you declare your diabetes on the application form, you may be asked about it at the interview. Many employers will know nothing at all about the illness, so you'll need to educate them. You may be asked if or how it is likely to affect your work. Be as honest as possible – if you need to inject insulin or take tablets while you're at work, just say, 'I may need a very short break to take my medication or to do a blood test.' If they're worried about you taking too much time off, explain that you're no more likely to take time off than someone who doesn't have diabetes (if this is true, of course – if you're in the habit of taking sickies, don't blame your diabetes or you'll cause problems for others!). Everybody is ill occasionally, and everyone needs to take time off for a hospital appointment now and again, as you will need to from time to time. You may have to make several appointments, for example with the consultant, the diabetes nurse and the dietician. If this is the case, try to arrange them all on the same morning so that the disruption to your job is minimal, and give your employer plenty of notice. And reassure him or her that studies have shown that most people with diabetes take no more time off than those who don't have diabetes.

The Disability Discrimination Act

Although you may not consider yourself disabled, the 1996 Disability Discrimination Act does extend to those with diabetes. Until recently, there were, in some areas of employment, restrictions on people whose diabetes was treated with insulin. This affected the police force, the fire service, people working at heights and people working off-shore, such as on oil rigs. There are still restrictions on some jobs that require the employee to drive. But in general, it is now against the law to discriminate against people with diabetes because of their diabetes. Before October 2004, this applied only to employers with 15 or more employees, but now, with the exception of the armed forces, it applies to all employers regardless of the size of the organization. This means that a person's fitness to work should be medically assessed, and if they are deemed fit, an employer who refused to employ them on the grounds of their diabetes would be breaking the law and may be liable under the Disability Discrimination Act. The Act also prevents employers

94

from sacking a member of their workforce who develops diabetes while in their employment. For more information on the Disability Discrimination Act, contact the Disability Rights Commission (see page 109).

Telling your colleagues

Whether you discuss your condition with your colleagues is something you'll need to think about. You may be reluctant because, as we have seen, there is a lot of ignorance about diabetes, and people who don't know anything about the disease can have some strange ideas and equally strange reactions. It's probably best to be quite 'matter-of-fact' about it, in the same way you would be if you had an allergy to something. Just explain the basics, tell them that you have to watch what you eat and that you have to take medication and test your blood regularly (if this is the case). If you're on insulin or other medication that can cause hypos, you should explain this to your colleagues as well, telling them what the symptoms are and what they should do if they spot the warning signs. Reassure them that, as your diabetes is well controlled, a hypo is fairly unlikely, but they should be aware that, occasionally, things can go wrong and a hypo may occur. Also, make sure you know who the designated first-aid person is and have a chat with that person about your condition as soon as possible.

Driving

Having diabetes doesn't necessarily mean you have to give up driving, but it may mean you have to take a little more care than someone who doesn't have diabetes, and you may need to renew your licence more often. Legally, you are obliged to inform the Driver and Vehicle Licensing Agency (DVLA) if your diabetes is treated with insulin, or if you have a relevant condition or complication (e.g. retinopathy) and your diabetes is treated with tablets. If you start off on diet alone and then move on to insulin, you need to tell them, as you do if you've been on tablets and a relevant related condition develops, or if you move from tablets to insulin. You don't need to tell them if you're on diet alone, but you must let them know if your condition or treatment changes.

If you are treated with insulin, you'll be issued with a licence for one, two or three years, and each time you renew it (renewal of restricted licences is free of charge) you'll be asked to fill in another form giving details of your diabetes and treatment. It's common sense really, but you absolutely must let them know if you develop any problems that affect your ability to drive. If you don't let them know, you may find that your insurance is no longer valid.

Poor eyesight due to retinopathy is obviously a potential problem and needs to be monitored. Neuropathy causing pain or loss of feeling is another example of a diabetes-related problem that can affect your driving, but perhaps the most serious problem is hypoglycaemia. If you are treated with insulin or with certain diabetes tablets, there is a risk that you may have a hypo, and if that were to happen while you were driving it could prove fatal, both for you and for other people. To avoid this, always keep some form of glucose with you, even when not driving. When you're in the car, make sure you have glucose tablets and biscuits, sandwiches or fruit that are easily accessible. Don't drive for more than two hours without stopping for a snack, check your blood glucose before and during a journey and be aware of the symptoms of hypoglycaemia. These include hunger, sweating, shakiness, palpitations, nausea, headache, faintness or dizziness. At the first sign of a hypo:

- Stop driving as soon as it is safe to do so and take glucose tablets, biscuits or other carbohydrate immediately.
- Leave the driving seat, remove the ignition key and step out of the car (if it's safe). This will refute any allegation that you were in charge of a car while under the influence of drugs (such as insulin).
- Don't set off again until you are completely recovered.
- If you have frequent hypos, or if you don't get sufficient warning signs that one is about to occur, you probably shouldn't be driving, and you should inform the DVLA. If you have an accident as a result of a hypo, you may be charged with driving under the influence of a drug, with driving without due care and attention or with dangerous driving. It is therefore vital to check your blood glucose levels before and during your journey to avoid this. If you do have a hypo while at the wheel, you should inform the DVLA. If they revoke your licence, you'll be able to appeal, but to win an appeal you must be able to convince them that the

episode was due to very unusual circumstances and that it is highly unlikely that you will have another hypoglycaemic attack while driving. If you have an accident due to a hypo, discuss what happened with your doctor, because if you genuinely believe a repeat occurrence is highly unlikely, your doctor's report may be very useful in an appeal situation.

Some points to remember:

- Notify the DVLA if you are on insulin or diabetes tablets.
- Also tell them if you have any related conditions or problems with your diabetes.
- Test your blood glucose levels before driving, and regularly if on a long drive.
- Avoid long or stressful journeys if you're tired.

Do not drive if:

- You have just started using insulin and your diabetes is not yet properly under control.
- You have difficulty recognizing the early warning signs of hypoglycaemia.
- You have any uncorrected problems with your eyesight.
- You have any numbness, tingling or weakness in your limbs due to neuropathy.

Travelling

As long as you're fairly fit and healthy, there's no reason why you shouldn't travel all over the world if you wish to. But whether you're travelling for business or pleasure, it's important to take your diabetes into account when planning your trip.

Travelling abroad

New security restrictions for aircraft travel mean that, if your diabetes is treated with insulin, you'll need to get a letter from your doctor confirming that you need to carry syringes or other injection devices while travelling. It may also be a good idea to carry some form of medical identification. Diabetes UK offers an insulin user's identity card, which has the user's name and photo, plus 'I have diabetes and am treated with insulin' written in English, French, Arabic, German and Spanish on the back. Contact Diabetes UK (see page 109) for an application form. The current price for the card is £5. It's a good idea to carry some form of medical ID, even when you're not travelling. Some people prefer to wear a special identification bracelet or necklace such as those available from the charity Medic Alert® (page 110).

When you are travelling by plane, your insulin needs to be packed in your hand luggage because it needs to be kept in the cabin as low temperatures in the hold may damage it. Remember that you may be asked to leave it with the cabin crew for them to store during the flight, so it's best to pack it in a separate carrier bag.

Make sure you find out in plenty of time whether you need to have vaccinations before travelling. Very occasionally, some 'live' vaccines can cause a reaction that results in a slight rise in blood glucose. If this happens and you take insulin, you may need to increase the dose for a short while – ask your health-care team for advice on what to do if this should happen. Most vaccines cause no problems at all.

If you should become ill while travelling, it's important to monitor your blood glucose levels frequently because illness can cause them to rise. You should continue with your insulin or diabetes tablets, even if you're not eating properly. If you can't face food, try replacing meals with soup or drinks of milk or fruit juice. If you have vomiting and diarrhoea, drink plenty of water to avoid dehydration, but also take regular sips of sugary drinks such as cola or lemonade (but not the diet versions). If you're in any way worried or unsure, seek medical advice.

Make sure you take extra tablets or insulin with you, just in case you become ill and need to increase your dose. Also, pack a spare set of equipment, just in case you and your luggage part company for any reason.

When arranging your travel insurance, check your policy to make sure that pre-existing conditions such as diabetes are not excluded. If the policy isn't clear, contact the insurers and ask them to confirm, in writing, that pre-existing conditions are not excluded in the event of you needing treatment, a hospital stay, emergency travel home or expenses for a prolonged stay due to illness.

Packing for the journey

Make sure you pack a supply of carbohydrate-rich foods in your hand luggage so that you can reach them easily. If you're on insulin or diabetes tablets and you're travelling by car, you should stop every two hours to test your blood glucose and have a snack if you need to. Be prepared – as well as planned snacks, have an emergency supply consisting of glucose tablets, cereal bars, fruit, biscuits, fruit juice and so on with you, just in case of traffic jams, delayed flights or buffet cars that run out of food. If your trip involves you crossing time zones, you may find you need an extra meal, together with extra insulin, or you may need to reduce your food intake and the amount of insulin. Have a chat with your diabetes care team about this before you travel. Many people pop back and forth across time zones with no problems at all, but it's as well to be prepared if there are problems.

Trains, planes and automobiles

Long periods of sitting still can cause circulation problems and swollen feet, so if possible, get up every half hour or so and have a wander down the aisle or carriage or, if you're travelling by car, try to stop fairly frequently to stretch your legs for a few minutes. Make sure you have comfortable shoes for the journey. If your feet are prone to swelling, take a larger size so that your shoes don't become too tight.

Hot weather

If you're travelling to a hot country, or even if you manage to time your British holiday with the one week of summer we seem to have in this country each year, beware of sunbathing! Not only will it give you wrinkles and increase your risk of skin cancer, but long periods of lying around doing nothing may raise your blood glucose levels, and if you have any numbness in your feet or legs, you may burn without noticing. This doesn't mean that you can't relax and enjoy a little sunshine – that's what a holiday is for, after all. But it does mean that you have to be even more vigilant than someone without diabetes.

Tips for coping with hot weather

- Use a high-factor sun protection cream. If you have numbness in your feet, protect them as you would protect your head, by keeping them covered where possible.
- If you've bought new shoes or sandals for your holiday, try them at home to make sure they fit and are comfortable. Don't walk around barefoot. When on the beach or swimming in the sea, wear plastic shoes or sandals in case of injury.
- Make sure you take a short walk or swim every so often to try and keep your blood glucose down.
- Drink plenty of water and sugar-free drinks to avoid dehydration.
- If you're on insulin, monitor your blood glucose regularly, because the hot weather can cause the insulin to be absorbed more quickly.
- Insulin can be damaged by very hot (or freezing) temperatures, and by bright light. Store your insulin in the fridge if there is one (not in the freezer compartment) or in a cool bag, as long as it doesn't come into contact with the ice packs. Or you could carry it in a cooled vacuum flask. Take insulin from its packaging and wrap in a wet cloth before placing in the flask.
- Diabetes UK produces a booklet called *Travel and Diabetes – Managing Away from Home*, which is packed with information and advice See page 109 for contact details.

Social life and eating out

In almost every culture, sharing meals with others is a pleasurable way of spending time with those who are dear to us and of bonding with people we don't know very well. We enjoy the food itself, the rituals surrounding the meal and the easy conversation around the table, whether it's Sunday lunch with the family or an elegant restaurant supper with friends. Major celebrations often have a meal at their heart – Christmas, New Year, Thanksgiving in the USA, weddings, christenings.

One of the things that people who have been newly diagnosed with diabetes worry about most is that they will no longer be able to enjoy these occasions because of restrictions on their diet. There's no point in pretending your diabetes is not going to make any difference to these occasions, because it is. You will clearly no longer be able to do the full turkey dinner with gravy, roast potatoes, bread sauce, cranberry jelly and three types of stuffing; not to mention the pre-lunch sherries, the Christmas pudding with brandy butter, the mince pies and the port and stilton to follow. But neither does it mean you have to sit there with a lettuce leaf and half a tomato. The more time and energy you're prepared to put into learning about healthy eating, the more choices you'll have when it comes to special meals. If you are entertaining at home, you'll be able to tailor the meals to suit your diet, but if you want to give your guests richer, higher-fat foods, simply change the sauce, dressing or accompaniments. For example, you could serve your guests poached salmon with hollandaise sauce, asparagus and new potatoes dripping in butter, and you could have salmon and asparagus with a generous squeeze of lemon, and maybe new potatoes tossed in a small amount of good quality olive oil with freshly ground black pepper and a hint of sea salt. While they have cream with their strawberries, you could have a little low-fat fromage frais. After a while, you'll start to love the clean, fresh taste of good food, simply cooked. By leaving off or modifying the 'extras', you can make a huge difference to the calorie, fat or sugar content of meals. Don't forget you can also have smaller portions – we all eat too much on special occasions, and most people can eat a lot less without even noticing it. If you get into the habit of having large portions of vegetables and salads and average portions of grilled chicken, poached fish, brown rice, bread or pasta, you can probably get away with the odd tiny portion of something naughty. Some people decide to have a taste of everything – just one mouthful. They say the first taste is usually the best anyway. That way, you can still have a tiny portion of many of the same things as your guests without jeopardizing your blood glucose levels. Much the same applies if you're in a restaurant or at a friend's house.

If you don't want your dining companions to know you have diabetes, or if your friends try to persuade you to eat things that you know are not good for you, say, I don't eat butter (or sugar or cream or whatever). It's harder to argue with that than with 'I can't eat . . .' or 'I'm on a diet' (when hearing that you're 'on a diet', many people see it as their mission to get you off it!). If they're trying to ply you with alcohol, you could always say you're driving, or you can't drink with the tablets you're taking. However, if they know you have diabetes and are still trying to tempt you off the straight and narrow, it may be that shock tactics are called for. It's overstating the case somewhat, but if they really won't accept what you say, tell them that eating that wedge of double chocolate fudge cake could seriously increase the risk that you might lose your sight or have to have your leg amputated. That should do the trick!

Tips for eating out or with friends

- Have a healthy snack before you go out so that you're not too hungry.
- Drink a glass of water before you eat – it'll make you feel fuller.
- Have two starters instead of a starter and a main course (many starters are lower in fat and carbohydrate than main courses – you may even be able to have three!).
- Take your own salad dressing.
- If you're with good friends, ask for a tiny taste of what they're having – you won't feel so deprived and you can join in with the rapturous compliments when your hosts serve something yummy.

New networks

Another positive thing about having diabetes is that you'll have plenty of opportunity to make new friends who know exactly what you're going through. There are a number of volunteer support groups throughout the country where you and your partner or other family members can go along and meet others who are living with diabetes. You can find details of your nearest group by contacting Diabetes UK (see page 109).

If you have access to the internet, you'll be able to join one of the many internet forums or newsgroups now available. You can become part of an on-line community, sharing concerns, information and ideas with others without ever having to leave your home. An internet newsgroup is like a bulletin board where people post messages. When you sign up, you'll be able to see the titles of messages other people have posted, and you can read those that interest you and post your own replies if you wish. Your replies can be read by everyone else, but your email address is kept private (unless, of course, you choose to disclose it to another user.) If you don't have internet access at home, you can use the computers at your local library (if you're not sure what to do, one of the library assistants should be able to help you).

The internet, incidentally, is a fantastic resource for learning more about your illness and keeping up to date with news of new treatments, book reviews and so on. A word of caution, however. Not everything you read on the internet is true, nor does it all come from reliable, genuine sources. Be especially suspicious of medicines that are sold over the internet, and bear in mind that, if a miracle cure is discovered, it'll probably be on national television or at the very least, on the websites of genuine diabetes organizations such as Diabetes UK or the American Diabetes Association. Some useful websites are listed in the Useful addresses section of this book (see page 109).

10

Myths and misconceptions

Most people are aware that there is an illness called diabetes, or 'sugar diabetes' as it used to be known, and that it affects quite a lot of people. But it's not until we are diagnosed ourselves or know someone else with the condition that we really start to understand it. Even then, unless you do a lot of reading on the subject, it's quite likely there will still be some things about it that are confusing or that you just don't know. As a result, there are a number of myths surrounding the illness, and this can lead to confusion, misunderstandings or even arguments, as explained here by Lucy, a 38 year-old teacher from Nottingham.

'I was diagnosed with type 2 diabetes three years ago,' says Lucy. 'It was a terrible shock – I'm not overweight, I'd hardly ever been ill as a child and I didn't even like sweet things. I was brought up by adoptive parents, so I suppose I must have inherited dodgy genes from my natural parents. I'm absolutely fine now, because I'm on insulin therapy and I'm very careful about remembering my medication, eating at the right times and so on and so forth.

'Anyway, one evening last term, I got delayed at the school parents' evening. It was the first one for the year sevens and of course their parents are all very concerned about how their sons are settling in their new school. I spent longer with each parent than I'd planned and although I'd started to feel hungry and a bit shaky, I stupidly didn't do anything about it. Then it suddenly dawned on me that my blood sugar was plummeting. I couldn't think straight, I broke out in a sweat and I felt faint. I knew I had to eat something quickly and I always keep a 'snack pack' of biscuits in my bag so that I can have one in an emergency. Knowing it would seem rather rude to just dive into my bag and start scoffing biscuits in front of my student and his parents, I said, "Excuse me, I'm diabetic and I need to eat." The next thing I knew, the boy's mother grabbed the packet from me yelling, "Stop! You can't eat that if you're diabetic!" It was nice that she was trying to help, but it made me really angry. When I explained, she apologized and said she thought it was dangerous for people with diabetes to have anything containing sugar.

'I'm sure she's not the only one to think that way, but I wish people would have the sense to realize that those of us who actually have the disease know what we're talking about when it comes to what we can and can't eat.'

True or false?

If you have diabetes, it is dangerous for you to eat biscuits, cakes or chocolate.

False. As Lucy's story shows, it is not dangerous and may even be appropriate as an emergency 'quick fix' if you feel your blood glucose levels falling. In general, semi-sweet biscuits are a better choice, and sweets, chocolate and other high-sugar items should be eaten sparingly, as part of a healthy meal.

Only fat people get type 2 diabetes

False. Although type 2 diabetes is much more common in those who are overweight (in fact, 80 per cent of people who are diagnosed with type 2 diabetes are overweight at the time of diagnosis), it also affects people of a healthy weight.

You can catch diabetes from someone else.

False. We don't know exactly why some people develop diabetes, but it is not contagious.

Type 2 diabetes can be prevented

True – we think! Many experts believe that controlling the diet and increasing exercise levels can prevent diabetes from developing. All are agreed that the onset can certainly be delayed.

Type 2 diabetes affects only middle aged and elderly people

False. One of the terms for type 2 diabetes used to be 'adult-onset' or 'mature-onset' diabetes because it was rarely seen in people under the age of 40 and was unusual in those under 50. This is no longer the case. The condition is becoming increasingly common in younger people, including adolescents and even younger children. This increased incidence is thought to be linked with the growing problem of obesity, particularly here and in the USA.

You get diabetes from eating too much sugar

False. This myth probably arises from the fact that you are more likely to develop type 2 diabetes if you are overweight, and you are more likely to be overweight if you eat a lot of sugary things such as cakes, biscuits and sweets.

You would know if you had diabetes

True AND false! Eventually of course, you will know you have type 2 diabetes. But one of the dangerous things about type 2 diabetes is that you can have it for months or even years without knowing. This is because the symptoms may initially be quite mild and you may confuse them with other health problems or simply put them down to the fact that you are getting older. If you think you may be at risk (see page 15), it would be sensible to ask your doctor for a test to make sure your blood glucose levels are normal.

It runs in families

True. If members of your family, especially first-degree relatives such as a parent or sibling, have either type 1 or type 2 diabetes, you are at greater risk of developing type 2. This is because your genetic make up means you are more prone to high blood glucose, either because your pancreas is not as efficient as it should be or because your body doesn't use insulin efficiently enough.

Diabetes is only serious if you need insulin

False. Diabetes is a serious, incurable illness. It is true that it can be well controlled with diet, exercise, tablets or insulin, or with a combination of these. It is also true that people with the disease can live long, happy, healthy lives. However, if blood glucose levels are not properly controlled, complications may develop. Some of these, including stroke and heart attack, can be fatal. Other serious complications include blindness, kidney failure, gangrene and amputation. This is why control of blood glucose levels when you have type 2 diabetes is vital.

If you have diabetes, you'll need to buy special diabetic foods

False. There is no need to spend money on special diabetic foods. A healthy diet for someone with type 2 diabetes is the same as a healthy diet for someone who doesn't have diabetes – low in fat, salt and sugar, and with plenty of wholegrain foods, loads of vegetables and two or three pieces of fruit. Diabetic foods still raise blood glucose levels, they can be quite expensive and some of them have a laxative effect.

Diabetes can make you go blind

True. Uncontrolled high blood glucose levels can damage parts of the eye causing permanent blindness. You're also more likely to develop cataracts, although these can be surgically removed if they seriously affect your vision.

If you have type 2 diabetes, you'll need to inject insulin for the rest of your life

False. People with type 1 need to take insulin, but if you have type 2, you may be able to control your diabetes with diet and exercise, certainly for a while. Some people are able to control their blood glucose this way for many years but find they need to take insulin eventually. See Chapter 7 for more information on insulin and how it is used.

You shouldn't play sports if you have diabetes

False. There is no reason at all why you shouldn't play sports. In fact, as explained in Chapter 6, regular physical activity can have a dramatic effect on your blood glucose levels and, combined with diet, can keep your diabetes under control and reduce your risk of developing complications.

Diabetes can lead to amputation

True. People with diabetes are more likely to suffer from gangrene, resulting in amputation. This is because prolonged raised blood glucose leads to decreased blood flow, especially to the legs and feet. An insufficient supply of blood to the body tissues can cause those tissues can die off. Gangrene is the name we give to this death of tissue. It can also be caused by infection of an open sore or ulcer. This is also more common in people with diabetes because nerve damage due to high blood glucose can cause loss of sensation in the feet. This means injuries to the foot may not be noticed until after infection has set in, and reduced blood flow may prevent the wound from healing properly.

You shouldn't drive if you have diabetes

False. There is no reason why you shouldn't drive, as long as you keep your blood glucose under control. Research has found that people with diabetes are no less safe on the roads than anyone else.

Useful addresses

British Complementary Medicine Association
PO Box 5122
Bournemouth
BH8 0WG
Tel.: 0845 345 5977
Website: www.bcma.co.uk
Email: info@bcma.co.uk

Diabetes UK
10 Parkway,
London NW10 7AA
Careline: 0845 120 2960
Tel.: 020 7424 1010 (customer services)
Website: www.diabetes.org.uk
Email: info@diabetes.org.uk

Disability Rights Commission
DRC Helpline
Freepost MID02164
Stratford-upon-Avon
CV37 9BR
Tel.: 08457 622633
Website: www.drc-gb.org

Driver and Vehicle Licensing Agency (DVLA)
Longview Road
Swansea
SA6 7JL
Tel: 0870 600 0301 (Drivers' Medical Section)
Website: www.dvla.gov.uk

Family Planning Association
2–12 Pentonville Road
London, N1 9FP

Helpline: 0845 310 1334 (9 a.m. to 6 p.m., Monday to Friday)
Website: www.fpa.org.uk

Limbless Association
Rehabilitation Centre
Roehampton Lane
London SW15 5PR
Tel.: 020 8788 1777
Website: www.limbless-association.org
Provides advice and information, plus a network of volunteer visitors (amputees themselves) to help those coming to terms with the loss of one or more limbs

Medic Alert®
1 Bridge Wharf
156 Caledonian Road
London N1 9UU
Tel.: 020 7833 3034
Freephone: 0800 581420
Website: www.medicalert.org.uk
Email: info@medicalert.org.uk

National Institute for Clinical Excellence (NICE)
71 High Holborn
London WC1V 6NA
Tel.: 020 7067 5800
Website: www.nice.org.uk
Email: nice@nice.org.uk

NHS direct
Tel: 0845 4647
Website: www.nhsdirect.nhs.uk

Royal National Institute of the Blind (RNIB)
105 Judd Street
London WC1H 9NE
Helpline: 0845 766 9999 (9 a.m. to 5 p.m., Monday to Friday)
Website: www.rnib.co.uk
Email: helpline@rnib.org.uk

Sexual Dysfunction Association
Windmill Place Business Centre
2–4 Windmill Lane
Southall,
Middlesex
UB2 4NJ
Helpline: 0870 7743571
Website: www.sda.uk.net
Email: info@sda.uk.net

Weight Watchers
Look in the phone book for local groups, or log on to:
www.weightwatchers.co.uk

Overseas organizations

American Diabetes Association
1701 North Beauregard Street
Alexandria
VA 22311
USA
Tel.: 001 800 342 2383
Website: www.diabetes.org

International Diabetes Federation
Avenue Emile De Mot 19
B-1000 Brussels
Belgium
Tel.: +32 2 5385511
Website: www.idf.org
Email: info@idf.org

Useful websites:

British Dietetic Association Weight Wise
www.bdaweightwise.com

For lots of easy-to-understand diabetes information and links to other American sites
www.mendosa.com/diabetes.htm

National Institute of Diabetes and Digestive and Kidney Diseases (USA)
www.niddk.nih.gov

Plymouth Library (prescription book scheme)
www.plymouth.gov.uk (click on 'leisure and tourism', then 'libraries' and follow link for information on the 'book prescription scheme')

Providing information on retinopathy
www.diabeticretinopathy.org.uk

Weight Concern
www.weightconcern.org.uk

Further reading

Becker, Gretchen. *Type 2 diabetes: the first year.* Robinson, 2004.

Blades, Mable, Jane Suthering and Antony Worral Thompson. *Antony Worral Thompson's GI diet.* Kyle Cathie, 2005.

Brewer, Sarah. *Natural approaches to diabetes.* Piatkus, 2005.

Carr, Allan. *Allan Carr's easy way to stop smoking.* Penguin, 1999.

Cutting, Derrick. *Stop that heart attack.* Class Publishing, 2004.

Day, J.L. *Living with diabetes: the Diabetes UK guide for those treated with diet and tablets only.* John Wiley and Sons, 2001.

Day, J.L. *Living with diabetes: the Diabetes UK guide for those treated with insulin.* John Wiley and Sons, 2003.

Drum, David Zierenberg and Terry. *The type 2 diabetes sourcebook.* Lowell House, 1998.

Fox, Charles, Sue Judd and Peter H. Sonsken (Foreword by Sir Steve Redgrave). *Diabetes at your fingertips.* Class Publishing, 2003.

Gilbert, Paul. *Overcoming depression.* Constable and Robinson, 2000.

Jovanovic-Peterson, Lois. *Managing your gestational diabetes: a guide for you and your baby's good health.* John Wiley and Sons, 1998.

Warshaw, Hope S. and Webb, Robyn. *The diabetes food and nutrition bible: a complete guide to planning, shopping, cooking and eating.* American Diabetes Association, 2001.

Also, *Balance Magazine* – six issues per year, produced by Diabetes UK.

Index